Narratives of Femicide Perpetrators in Latin America

Martín Hernán Di Marco

Narratives of Femicide Perpetrators in Latin America

Taking Lives

palgrave
macmillan

Martín Hernán Di Marco
Institute of Security and Global Affairs
(ISGA)
Leiden University
The Hague, The Netherlands

ISBN 978-3-031-97366-6 ISBN 978-3-031-97367-3 (eBook)
https://doi.org/10.1007/978-3-031-97367-3

Cover illustrations: Lorena Leonhardt
Inside illustrations/Figures: Laura Spangenberg

This Palgrave Macmillan imprint is published by the registered company Springer Nature Switzerland AG
The registered company address is: Gewerbestrasse 11, 6330 Cham, Switzerland

To the women whose voices were silenced.

To my mum, whose strength and unwavering spirit inspire me to seek understanding in even the most complex of human stories.

And to Morten, who has shown me new ways of loving.

Foreword

If we were to cast the role of a man who kills his intimate partner, many would conjure the image of Gaston. You know the one. The broad-chested brute from *Beauty and the Beast*. He swaggers through the town, flexing, bellowing, throwing back tankards of ale. He farts. He yells. He commands. And in his mind, protagonist Belle belongs to him. He believes he is entitled to her beauty, her affection, her body, simply because he is a man. There is nothing ambiguous about Gaston. He is violence before it has even been committed. He is a walking, belching warning sign. And yet, the men in this book are not Gaston.

This book reveals a different truth, a harder, messier truth. The nine men whose stories unfold in these pages are not caricatures of aggression. They do not stomp into rooms demanding obedience. They are not cartoonishly evil, nor are they, in all cases, obvious threats. They are fathers, husbands, boyfriends. They are quiet, polite, thoughtful even. They hold jobs. They have friends. They are more than the worst thing they have done, and yet, that worst thing—killing their intimate partner—is an undeniable, irreversible fact.

There is an impulse, a very human one, to make sense of femicide by categorising its perpetrators. If we can define them, we can locate them, and if we can locate them, perhaps we can stop them. We like the idea of a prototype: the abuser who escalates, the controlling partner who isolates, the jealous man who seethes. In many cases, those patterns exist, but they do not tell the full story.

The truth is that femicide is not always predictable. It does not always present itself in raised voices, broken plates, or bruises hidden beneath long sleeves. It does not always come with clenched fists or snarled insults. Sometimes it comes from the man who was never violent before. The one who seemed fine. The one no one suspected. That is the discomfort at the heart of this book. If femicide had a prototype, we could intervene with certainty. But instead, we are left with complexity, contradiction, and a difficult question: how do we stop violence when its perpetrators do not always look violent?

Martín's work emphasises the role of perpetrators' own storytelling and their relationship to cultural discourses in femicides. For instance, when he identifies different narrative structures that run through the stories of these otherwise highly unalike perpetrators. Against a backdrop of fear of loss or betrayal, infidelity and abandonment, these men often feel justified retaking their male authority. Social or cultural factors, such as upbringing or societal expectations, often work as excuses for the crimes they committed. Moreover, frequent attempts were made to silence victims, and victims' concerns described as overreactions, reinforcing isolation and suppressing dissent. Referring to a shared understanding of masculinity and emphasising support from peers was similarly crucial. Many of the men also saw themselves as victims and downplayed the violence they had committed.

In all these stories, there is a fine line between the stories of those that have committed femicides and the language of the broader machismo culture in Latin American societies. Martín has a hopeful proposition of change, describing how the young men talked differently and less assertively about their violence than the older men—and described less peer support than their elders. At the same time, with the recent growth of the online "manosphere" normalised through public figures like Andrew Tate and supported by social media algorithms, one can fear that such positive changes are only temporary and already a thing of the past.

This book delves into the narratives of men who have committed intimate femicide in Latin America, offering a unique lens through which to understand the underlying motivations and societal structures that perpetuate this form of violence. By examining the life stories of these perpetrators, this text uncovers the cultural context as well as the social narratives that sustain such acts. Femicide is not merely a series of isolated incidents but a reflection of deeply ingrained gender norms and power dynamics that manifest in extreme violence.

Martín's work offers several important contributions to a multitude of research fields, and there are both empirical and theoretical lessons to be learned for everyone. Readers will find different parts of it interesting, and the presentations of lengthy cases allows for numerous associations and connections, possibly reaching far beyond the author's own interpretations. As scholars in criminology, narrative studies, and public health, we emphasise the contributions to the research areas that we are most familiar with.

In recent years, research on intimate partner homicide has mostly focused on prevalence, warning signs, typologies, and the roles of mental and behavioural disorders among intimate partner homicide perpetrators. While this work is crucial, Martín takes a different path. He delves into the stories perpetrators tell—how they frame their actions, how cultural narratives shape their justifications, and how identity plays a role in these crimes. By giving perpetrators an in-depth voice, he exposes the ways in which they construct meaning around their violence. This is difficult, necessary work, adding nuance to the study of femicide and deepening our understanding of the forces that drive it.

Secondly, revealing how closely linked storytelling is to harmful action, the book is an exemplary case and great contribution to narratives studies in general and narrative criminology in particular. Martín moves this nascent research field forward by linking a study of the most archetypical crime—the killing of another person—to classics in narrative studies from both the humanities and the social sciences. The emphasis on overarching recognisable contents of these stories, as well as the different story structures, and the link of both to more general cultural stories is nothing but impressive. The overall project of linking storytelling to harmful action is at the core of narrative criminology. The depth, originality and clear-sightedness make the book a must-read for anyone in this or related research traditions—or for just anyone interested in narrative theory and research.

Finally, femicide, the killing of women and girls due to their gender, is a profound public health crisis that demands urgent attention and action. The public health perspective emphasises the need to address these root causes through a multifaceted approach that includes prevention, intervention, and policy reform. These perpetrators narratives provide valuable insights into the social and psychological factors that drive such violence, highlighting the importance of early intervention and the promotion of healthy, equitable relationships. By exploring the stories of men who have committed femicide, we can identify patterns and commonalities that inform targeted prevention efforts, ultimately aiming to reduce the incidence of such violence and save lives.

In presenting these narratives, this book challenges prevailing stereotypes and offers a nuanced understanding of femicide. In line with narrative research and theorising the emphasis is not on the individual, but on the collective and social dimension of the stories that makes evil possible. In keep with principles of public health and homicide studies, it calls for a shift in focus from responsive or punitive measures to preventive strategies that address the underlying individual *and* social determinants driving the phenomenon. By examining the structural factors that contribute to femicide, we can develop more effective interventions that not only respond to violence but also work to prevent it from occurring in the first place.

Martín's work does not offer easy answers, because there are none. Instead, he presents the foundational *stories* justifying, motivating, fueling, and even arousing femicide, in all their nuance and complexity. He asks us to look beyond the Gaston-like brute, beyond the obvious villain. Not to sympathise. Not to excuse. But to understand how the stories of femicide perpetrators are intertwined and embedded in widespread stories about gender, relationships, and love. When the Argentine bolero performer Cacho Castaña sings *Si te agarro con otro te mato* (If I Find You with Another Man, I'll Kill You), as Martín writes, this reflects widespread narratives about love, violence, and control that goes way beyond people who commit femicide. Because only in understanding the links between the individual men and the narrative environment facilitating such crimes can we begin to change the story.

Atlanta, USA — Prof. Dabney P. Evans
The Hague, The Netherlands — Prof. Marieke Liem
Oslo, Norway — Prof. Sveinung Sandberg

Preface

I began this book as an effort to bring closure and consolidate the material I had collected over six years of research. In the process, I found myself juggling three potential versions of a manuscript: an academic book advocating for a narrative approach to understanding violence, an attempt to engage a broader audience with a non-individualising explanation of these violent offences, and a reflection on femicide and societal change over time.

My aim here is to reinvigorate a debate that, in my view, has become somewhat stagnant—often reduced to clichés, vague concepts, and an oversimplified understanding of risk factors. I also hope to draw readers closer to the everyday realities we often hear about, choose to ignore, reproduce inadvertently, but rarely challenge. By focusing on this diffuse and intangible aspect of society—the system of stories that structure our worldviews—I believe we can contribute to preventing this form of violence.

One of the main challenges I faced while writing was deciding on a single style and structure, as this meant leaving other possible approaches behind. Initially, I sought to break away from traditional academic prose and write in the style of a chronicle. However, I eventually gravitated back to a more academic format, partly due to inertia. In the style I have chosen—which aligns with the traditions of qualitative social sciences—I aim to be accessible to readers from diverse backgrounds. The decision to include vignettes in the form of short relationship biographies serves as a device to provide non-specialist readers with an entry point into the topic, avoiding the rigidity of other formats.

Another significant challenge was the emotional toll of writing this book. Many colleagues asked about the emotional labour involved in interviewing men who had killed, assuming that this aspect was particularly taxing or even threatening. However, I found the contextual challenges of the post-fieldwork phase to be far more demanding. Writing on the move, changing academic positions and countries, and witnessing my home country, Argentina, descend into institutional chaos and economic uncertainty were all deeply unsettling. I also encountered the harsh realities of hostile academic audiences, vicious criticism, and blind rivalry. In light of recent critiques of extractivism in the social sciences—where researchers mine data from vulnerable communities without meaningful engagement or reciprocity—and internal tensions within the field of violence against women, I feel it is important to acknowledge these discomforts as part of being honest about my crossroads standpoint while writing this book.

Finally, I hope this book avoids falling into what Bourgois (2003) once referred to as the pornography of violence: representing it in a sensationalised, fetishised way at the expense of deeper structural explanations. While the discomfort elicited by the description of perpetrators' stories is undeniable, I believe it remains essential to delve into the logics underpinning their violent acts—confronting the issue directly and addressing it with clarity and honesty.

Ultimately, if you are seeking a book that offers definitive answers, prioritising a 'demand for answers' over the 'quest for meaning' (Lacan, 1973), this may not be the right choice for you. And if such an analysis—prioritising complexity over quick answers—remains difficult to grasp in 2025, more than a century after the emergence of interpretative sociology, perhaps it suggests that we are still struggling with deep-seated structural issues in our ways of understanding the social world.

The Hague, The Netherlands

Martín Hernán Di Marco

Acknowledgements Every book is, inevitably, a collective endeavour. This is not merely a gesture of political correctness but a reflection of the process itself. The institutions and individuals mentioned below, as well as those I may have inadvertently overlooked, provided material, intellectual, or emotional support that made the research underpinning this book possible.

I begin by addressing the foundational aspects of this book: its material conditions. This study was made possible through funding from The Research Council of Norway (RCN) under the Crime in Latin America—CRIMLA project (NFR 324299), which explores the role of the state, labour market, family, culture, and religion in crime in Latin America. Additional support was provided by the Department of Criminology and Sociology of Law (IKRS) at the University of Oslo, which contributed to cover art, illustrations, proofreading costs, and an endless supply of coffee within a supportive environment. Initial funding was also provided by the Faculty of Social Sciences (FSOC) at the University of Buenos Aires through their Proyecto de Reconocimiento Institucional (PRI) programme (Res. DAR 2938/20), awarded to me in 2020. Finally, the Femicide Perpetration Pooled Data Project at the Rollins School of Public Health, Emory University, played a helpful role in consolidating this extensive dataset. As this book was written during a new wave of neoliberal dismantling of the Argentine state, including its science sector, these funds were not merely a crucial incentive but indispensable for its completion.

The core group of people with whom I discussed this manuscript and ideas included Sveinung Sandberg and Dabney P. Evans. Sveinung, alongside Gustavo Fondevila, led the CRIMLA project and served as a guiding mentor in narrative criminology. Having one of the founding scholars of this field inspire this text has been invaluable. Dabney has been my academic mentor and collaborator over the past six years, with our shared interest in violence perpetration. Her insightful guidance has been pivotal in navigating the often nebulous field of violence studies—where journals from different disciplines continue to debate who should 'dominate' the niche, and grant evaluators still struggle to recognise the importance of understanding aggressors. Her support has been truly indispensable.

I completed most of the book during my postdoctoral fellowship at the Department of Criminology and Sociology of Law at the University of Oslo. This experience was enriching for me, and I hope this is reflected in the following pages. I am grateful to all the scholars who generously read manuscripts, engaged in discussions on the ideas expressed in the book, or patiently listened to my musings over *matpakke*. Special thanks are due to the invaluable support of Anja Emilie Kruse, Eva Magdalena Stambøl, My Rafstedt, Pernille Nyvoll, Randi Solhjell, Rose Elisabeth Lunde, and Stefano Mazzilli Daechsel. Sophia Angelis kindly reviewed the book proposal when we had just met. Finally, Helene Oppen Ingebrigtsen Gundhus supported this project from the beginning and provided additional resources, actually making it a viable endeavour.

The Red Interamericana Anti Femicidio (RIAF) has been an ambitious initiative aimed at connecting researchers, activists, practitioners, and policymakers addressing femicide across the Americas. The discussions held in RIAF surrounding the uses (and misuses) of academic knowledge in the field of violence against women reshaped my understanding of knowledge production.

The International Sociological Association (ISA) provided a fertile space for learning about sociological discussions on biographies and violence across different countries. The Research Committee 38 'Biography and Society' and Working Group 11 'Violence and Society', in which I still hold institutional positions, offered a breath of fresh air for collective reflection and a commitment to a sociological understanding of this topic. I am particularly grateful to Myrna Dawson and Sylvia Walby from Working Group 11, and Johannes Becker from Research Committee 38, for their support.

Additionally, the Community of Practice for the Study of Domestic Homicide (CoPSDH) has been an invaluable space for exchanging ideas with other scholars and practitioners working in the field of homicide, particularly in the United Kingdom. Special thanks to John Devaney, James Rowlands, and Stephanie Holt.

The Global Qualitative Sociology Network, conceived by Marian Burchardt and Johannes Becker, served me as a pivotal forum for discussion. I presented initial ideas from the book and received invaluable feedback. I am particularly grateful to Eva Bahl, Soledad Balerdi, Hilal Alkan, and Weishan Huang for their comments during our workshop in La Plata in the summer of 2023.

Three subsequent research projects (CYTMA2 from the Universidad Nacional de La Matanza), which I led, fostered an inspiring process of reflection on gender-based violence and discourse. I am deeply grateful to my co-leader and friend, Adrián Jiménez Ribera, for his tireless enthusiasm, and to the entire team for their patience: Florentina Cavaro, Magalí Brizuela, María Florencia Santi, and Wanda Cabrera. This would not have been possible without the financial support of the Department of Health Sciences, under the leadership of Graciela Brito and Mariela Ferrari.

I would also like to thank Juan Antonio Rodriguez for generously sharing his data and for his unwavering encouragement. James Rowlands provided crucial feedback throughout the process. Laura Spangenberg brilliantly created the chapter illustrations, while Lorena Leonhardt skilfully designed the cover art. Alba Font Cuadras, Esther Nakano, and Esmée Turpijn, enthusiastic master's students at Leiden University, conducted a thorough read-through of the manuscript and provided feedback.

In the process of writing, I shared drafts and comments with several individuals who provided feedback and helped decide on the artwork. My heartfelt thanks to Ana Castiglione, Anahi Sy, Anja E. Kruse, Ardath Whynacht, Claire Branigan, Dabney P. Evans, Elizabeth Dartnall, Evangelina Caravaca, Fira Chmiel, Gabriela Cormick, Gustavo Fondevila, Helena Suárez Val, Johannes Becker, John Devaney, Krzysztof Strąk, Lizle Loots, Marie Bessieres, My Rafstedt, Myrna Dawson, Paula Malzone, Rosario Figari Layús, Sine Holen, Solveig Laugerud, and, of course, my mum, Diana Mutti.

Upon completing this book, I began my new position as Assistant Professor at the Institute of Security and Global Affairs (ISGA) at Leiden University. My new research group was not only welcoming but also kind enough to allow me to present the core ideas and points of this book. Special thanks to Marieke Liem, Mischa Dekker, Jolien van Breen, Katharina Krüsselmann, Olga Bogolyubova, Laura van Gunst, Layla van Wieringen, and Kamilla Haugen.

Special thanks also go to the dedicated researchers who contributed to conducting part of the interviews, especially Liza Zúñiga Collado, Magalí Quispe, and Luis Enrique Amaya. Their commitment to the research process was crucial to the success of this project.

I also dedicate this work to everyone working with and supporting the Sexual Violence Research Initiative (SVRI) and their monumental efforts in preventing violence against women and children. Your commitment is admirable.

I must also acknowledge the material and geopolitical context in which this book was written. Having lived in four countries and changed academic positions three times during its development highlights two key issues. First, the precariousness of academic positions, where securing funding often consumes as much time as research itself, making our work both challenging and unstable. Second, most of the funds for this research came from the Global North, raising questions about how the uneven distribution of resources affects our research agendas. It is worth considering whether this book would have been possible or completed with Latin American funding. These issues deserve our critical attention.

* * *

Anti-Acknowledgement Finally, I wish to offer my acknowledgements in an unconventional manner. Alongside my work with men who have committed homicide, I have also encountered tensions and contradictions embedded in academic spaces that present themselves as progressive. At times, I observed dynamics—from the marginalisation of colleagues and the reproduction of gendered hierarchies, to cultivating hostile workplaces—that stood in stark contrast to those professed ideals. These patterns, often met with institutional silence, have informed and deepened my understanding of harm. While direct experience is not a prerequisite for *verstehen*, the reflections in this book are shaped in part by the complexities of witnessing and navigating such environments.

Competing Interests The author has no competing interests to declare that are relevant to the content of this manuscript.

Contents

About the Author

Martín Hernán Di Marco is an Assistant Professor in the Violence and Violence Prevention Research Group at the Institute of Security and Global Affairs (ISGA), Faculty of Governance and Global Affairs, Leiden University, Netherlands. He holds a B.A. in Sociology from the University of Buenos Aires, an M.Sc. in Epidemiology, Management, and Health Policies from the National University of Lanús, and a Ph.D. in Social Sciences from the University of Buenos Aires, Argentina. He completed his postdoctoral appointment at the Institute of Criminology and Sociology of Law (IKRS) at the University of Oslo, Norway. Additionally, he serves as an Adjunct Professor at the Rollins School of Public Health, Emory University, USA.

During the writing of this book, he worked on the Crime in Latin America (CRIMLA) project at the University of Oslo (RCN 324299) and the Narratives of Life and Death project (PRI DAR No. 2938) at the Faculty of Social Sciences, University of Buenos Aires.

List of Figures

Part I

Setting the Stage

1

Introduction

Femicide, Perpetrators and Their Stories

I began speaking with Yoel in 2017. He was 47 years old and had been incarcerated three and a half years earlier for the femicide of his wife. We had first met several months prior at a prison event where university lecturers were allowed to attend. After a series of conversations over the following month, he agreed to share what he referred to as "his side of the story". Like many of the men I interviewed, he was deeply concerned about how others perceived the crime he had committed:

– Yoel: People just think you go mental, or that you're some monster, viciously torturing your wife with a rolling pin for years or something. Or that you hate women [smirks], like, all the women in the world! Or that you've always been mental, completely fucked up. But the truth is, no one can know what happens except the two of us. Outsiders have no say. The media? They talk a load of bollocks, they just want to sell. The judges? They're all grabbed by the balls and desperate to be politically correct for the feminazis. And now this is femicide [stresses]! What the fuck even is femicide? Killing someone because of their gender? You don't kill someone because of their gender

M. H. Di Marco, *Narratives of Femicide Perpetrators in Latin America*, https://doi.org/10.1007/978-3-031-97367-3_1

[stresses], whatever that even means. Explain to me how that works. You might end up in a fight, completely driven by love or frustration, and things just go wrong. That's not because of gender [stresses]. That's an accident, something that happens because of the history of the re-la-tion-ship [draws out syllables].

- Martín: A relationship.
- Y: Aha. I know this is not a popular opinion, but that's how things were for us. Not a fucked-up relationship, not an unstable guy stalking his young, sexy neighbour. Just a couple with difficulties and things going out of control. [...] No one even talks about her. How she loved to create frustration, to push me over the edge. I bet if the situation was the other way around, things would be different.
- M: Different?
- Y: It would have probably been self-defence. I bet on it. My lifelong best friend, from all my life, testified. He told everyone how she pushed me, she pushed me. And even though he's criticised me for loads of stuff, he stands by my side and says this is a huge misunderstanding.

Yoel's account was filled with self-defence and a strong desire to present a morally sound persona. However, in contrast to other men convicted of homicide, his story included more elements of righteousness connected to larger topics like state policy and social movements. Clearly, femicide was a topic at the centre of the storm, compelling him to address more than just interpersonal matters.

When I conducted this interview, my focus was not specifically on stories about femicide. The conversation stemmed from a project on homicide, but my curiosity was peaked. Over the years, as I began to delve into the field of intimate partner violence, I realised that Yoel's account bears many similarities to those of other men I would later interview across the Latin American countries where I conducted fieldwork and accessed data. He challenged the interpretation of femicide, disputing the notion that gender was the primary motive. He also provided an emphatic rationalisation of the homicide, separating the prior violence from the killing itself, which he portrayed as an isolated event, almost suspended in time. Additionally, he attempted to cast himself in a more favourable light by depicting his wife as the instigator. As the narration unfolded, he shifted from speaking in the first person (I) to using the impersonal pronoun (one). Most notably, he introduced his "lifelong best" friend into the narrative to support his account: while his friend had criticised him, he also expressed a degree of support.

In the years following my interview with Yoel, news of other homicides of women increasingly appeared in the media across Latin America with the rise of *Ni Una Menos*. Although this was not a new issue, it was certainly gaining traction in the public sphere, evolving in both scope and intensity. Within these discussions, no single narrative emerged to describe these men: some were portrayed as having an 'aggressive personality disorder', others as 'psychopaths' or 'narcissists'. Some were seen as 'embodiments of patriarchy', exhibiting a pattern of controlling behaviour, while in some cases, they were simply labelled as 'monsters'. Tied to these discourses—although not necessarily in a coherent manner—were some secondary discussions about how to deal with the perpetrators. Some called for harsher sentencing, while others advocated for upstream policies, like mental health assessments from an earlier age, or wider public engagement with the issue.

Journalists were not the only actors providing images about these men. Television series and films from the 2000s also provided perspectives on homicides of women and the men involved. These stories played a key role in shaping the broader imagination surrounding the topic. A wave of literary depictions across genres also fuelled the conversation, including *Siempre será después* (Schultze, 2012) from Uruguay and *Conchita* (Palacios, 2016) from Argentina. In the following years, a steady flow of books reinforced this trend: *Los divinos* (Restrepo, 2018) from Colombia, *La fosa del agua* (Carrión, 2018) and *El invencible verano de Liliana* (Rivera Garza, 2021) from Mexico, *Cometierra* (Reyes, 2019) from Argentina, and *The simple art of killing a woman* (Melo, 2023) from Brazil. From the North, television series such as *The Fall*, *The Staircase*, and *The Undoing* also signalled the increasing awareness—and commercialisation—of the topic.

All these cultural products helped to set the tone regarding cases of women and girls being killed because of their gender. They contributed to creating the general narrative reality in which elements of Latin American societies thought about and discussed these crimes. Naturally, they were not the only discursive offerings addressing the issue: decades of feminist mobilisation, culminating in *Ni Una Menos*, had raised public awareness of violence against women in Latin America (Lagarde y de los Ríos, 2012). Later, these proclamations were translated into the legal language of the state in many countries (Pasinato & de Ávila, 2022). More broadly, states, third-sector organisations, family advocacy groups and activists incorporated new terms and approaches into their efforts, calling for 'due diligence in femicide investigations' and emphasising state responsibility in prosecuting these crimes. Yet, few discourses delved into the mindset of the men who committed these crimes.

Grasping the motivations behind a violent act is no straightforward task. Since the inception of the social sciences, researchers have grappled with the complex nexus between meaning, action, and context. From Max Weber onwards, a longstanding tradition of scholars has emphasised the need to decode the perceived rationality of an action, as understood (and explained) by those directly involved. In essence, understanding rationality involves focusing on social actions guided by calculation, rules, or values, which shape behaviour and contribute to a particular worldview. However, in an era of growing fascination with violence (Binik, 2020) and its conceptual inflation (Noel & Garriga Zucal, 2010), where countless readily digestible explanations have been fabricated, this endeavour has become even more challenging. What drove these men to act in such a way? Is it as straightforward as the media suggests? Or do they possess such a dark, deranged quality that it defies logical comprehension? And are there shared motives among perpetrators? A range of discourses—from tabloid journalism and oversimplified TV scripts to slogan-driven activist narratives—promote superficial answers to these questions. Meanwhile, murder is "enjoyed and consumed" as a social product (Worsley, 2014, p. 2).

In this evolving context, I find myself questioning the rationality of the men who committed these crimes. This is driven by the paradox that David Riches (1986) highlighted decades ago, and it remains relevant today: while many actors talk about violence, we rarely inquire into how perpetrators themselves talk about it. This has been a pivotal idea that has driven the development of numerous lines of inquiry, yet we—as academics and as a society—still struggle to adopt this approach when dealing with certain crimes like sexual abuse, paedophilia, and homicide.

This book delves into the stories of men who have been convicted of murdering their intimate partners in seven Latin American countries. More specifically, it seeks to understand the stories they use to make sense of their past experiences, intimate relationships, friendships, turning points, and, ultimately, the act of murder itself. While gruesome, it is as straightforward as that. This exploration is grounded in, and aims to contribute to, the relatively recent field of narrative criminology (Presser & Sandberg, 2015). My aim is to steer the conversation away from one dominated by individualising explanations—such as psychological labelling detached from social contexts—, isolated risk factors, reductive tropes like jealousy as a trigger, or overly rigid structural concepts that flatten a textured understanding of violence and its evolution. Instead, I aim to foster more culturally informed discussions. With this book I argue that, if we are to understand, theorise, and ultimately prevent the systematic killing of women and girls, we must explore the narratives that underpin such actions. These harrowing stories might be pronounced by individuals, but they are shaping—and shaped by—broader structural forces within our society.

This book presents four main empirically grounded arguments. First, across Latin America, narratives sustaining femicide often revolve around the violation of gender norms, with violence used instrumentally to address perceived infractions. This justice-seeking action forms part of a broader narrative arc that highlights the importance of rule-breaking in the perpetuation of violence. The second argument emphasises that femicide cannot be fully understood without considering the surrounding contexts—stories of friendships, family dynamics, and impunity. These interconnected narratives reveal how intimate femicides unfold within a wider social fabric. Third, the book explores how social contexts are embedded in perpetrators' narratives. Even when these accounts may be dismissed as outliers or easily labelled with psychiatric diagnoses, the same overarching themes—entitlement, punishment, expectation, perceived harm persist across stories. Finally, the book observes a generational shift in the way perpetrators of femicide narrate their actions.

Younger offenders describe their violence with less impunity, diminished victim-blaming, and reduced social support, indicating a shift in societal attitudes. These evolving stories offer a glimpse into a changing cultural landscape that aligns with the declining rates of femicide in the region.

By presenting these arguments through narrative vignettes, this book pieces together an alternative to the facile explanations of intimate femicide that have taken root over the past three decades. Broad foundational concepts, such as patriarchy and coercive control, have guided our research, activism, advocacy, and even policy design. Despite their merits, these concepts have congealed into a *doxa*—though originally formed as a form of counter-discourse—which has tended to oversimplify the multifaceted nature of the phenomenon, as Bendelli (2017) has argued. Much like what has occurred with the notion of 'rape culture' (Bumiller, 2008; Whynacht, 2019), these concepts-turned-lay terms have inevitably oversimplified discussions, erasing the complexities and nuances of intimate partner violence.

The approach I have chosen involves examining the narrative landscape through the first-hand accounts of perpetrators themselves. I ground my perspective in the diverse field of perpetrator studies and the social study of narratives. My focus is on storytelling and how men's accounts link them to a broader discursive reality, particularly in Latin America. Exploring these interconnected narratives is far from a superficial endeavour. As Presser (2013, p. 25) argues, by "taking discourse seriously", we can observe how the ways in which we remember, make sense of our interactions and experiences, and uphold expectations, contribute to harmful actions, regardless of the factual accuracy of these stories.

However, this book is not a critique of how we arrived at our current level of awareness and mobilisation. Instead, it is an attempt to unsettle the impression that everything has been said about femicide and its causes. While this prevailing doxa is undoubtedly reassuring—as a milestone in changing gender norms—it may also act as a constraint, limiting a critical and nuanced understanding of what patriarchy and risk factors truly entail.

Ultimately, my goal is to anchor this study in a profound understanding of the logic behind intimate femicide. In doing so, I also explore the flipside of mainstream discussions surrounding the conditioning factors of femicide: I seek to provide subjective meanings to the triggers and factors, such as separation and jealousy. As Mary Douglas (1992) famously argued, risk is not merely a measure of danger or probability; it is also a reflection of the meanings we attach to particular hazards. Understanding risk factors requires us to engage with the cultural systems that shape our perceptions. This approach requires us to move beyond the idiosyncrasies of any one particular Latin American country. For this reason, I have selected cases that vary in age, educational and occupational trajectories, and neighbourhoods. Thus, life stories serve not only as the textual material of analysis but also as a prism through which to connect perpetrators across the region.

The title of this book, *Taking Lives*, reflects both the nature of my research and its implications. On one hand, the act of taking the lives of women is the central focus of my inquiry, which unites the men I interviewed. On the other hand, my writing process involved deliberately taking fragments of their lives and arranging them to reveal some of the most prevalent analytical issues that I believe are key to deciphering femicides.

While the opening quotes from Yoel's interview were particularly stark and blunt—almost archetypally direct in its victim-blaming—they serve as a fitting starting point for this book, condensing some key elements present in most interviews. I deliberately omitted his nationality, as a prelude to the approach I will take. The fact that not all interviewees were as confrontational or addressed precisely the same topics, yet expressed similar views on the crime, provides a foundation for exploring the narratives that underpin this form of violence in Latin America.

Book Structure

This book is divided into three parts.

Part I outlines the aim and foundations of this work. Following this Introduction, Chapter 2, *Why?*, establishes the reasoning and motivations behind the overall endeavour. I make the case not only for the usefulness of understanding the rationalities underpinning intimate femicides but also for how the lack of such research has misled current scholarly discussions.

Chapter 3, *What?*, focuses on some of the central theoretical coordinates of the narrative approach to perpetrators. The aim here is to ease the reader into the hermeneutic perspective of the book, and to provide an overview of how narratives work in societies.

Chapter 4, *How?*, offers a detailed description of how the fieldwork was conducted and how fieldwork and ethical dilemmas were addressed throughout the research. Overall, this chapter is intended to help readers understand the practical aspects of the study.

Part II comprises the vignettes of the men interviewed. The chapters in this section are presented as narratives, deliberately combining the men's own words with my reconstruction of their stories. This approach aims to foreground the main arguments, narrative arcs, and key features of their accounts in a manner that, while informed by analytical categories, avoids overwhelming the text with excessive interpretation. This part is organised around three analytical aspects, each increasing in complexity: safeguarding the status quo, social networks and institutions, and finally, social contexts and 'off' narratives. The chapters are arranged to reflect this progression.

In Chapter 5, I present three life stories that illustrate how men's perceptions of the status quo are key to understanding their aggression. Jorge, Celso, and Héctor share a deeply ingrained sense of moral boundaries. In their narratives, they reconstruct how breaches of certain social norms—such as domesticity, fidelity, and loyalty—constituted direct threats to them as men. Violating the status quo triggered a dissolution of their sense of self, revealing the implicit moral rules governing intimate relationships.

In Chapter 6, I present three vignettes that broaden the picture of intimate femicide. These stories show that such crimes are not confined to a victim-perpetrator dyad. The accounts of Matías, João, and José foreground the roles of friends, neighbours, and institutions in either enabling, concealing, or ignoring male violence. These narratives underscore the broader web of actors, institutions, and places implicated in these crimes.

In Chapter 7, I examine how men interpret their own acts of harm and how their narratives either weave in or omit social contexts. These accounts, regardless of how easily they can be framed in psychological or medical terms, provide a basis for understanding femicide. Alberto frames his actions within a broader context of societal change, expressing feelings of being overwhelmed by "feminazis" and a loss of agency, while also reflecting the influence of therapeutic and institutional discourses on life story reconstruction. Hugo, by contrast, erases social context, presenting the femicide as an isolated event driven by his wife's actions and his own indifference towards others. Lastly, Aldemar's fragmented narrative, while suggestive of schizophrenia, exposes deeper contextual factors and entrenched misogyny.

Part III provides an interpretation of the life stories discussed in the previous chapters and delves into the underlying patterns of the narratives across Latin America.

Chapter 8 explores common aspects in the stories of perpetrators, forming a moral economy of stories that sustain femicide. Themes include the disruption of gender norms, the clash of tacit expectations, the normalisation and embodiment of control. This chapter also argues that supportive narratives—from friends, inoperative neighbours, and complicit institutions—are necessary complements to stories solely focused on violence against women. These narratives create a broader web of interconnected stories (not all directly about violence or women), forming a *tessellated* structure. Violence, as a legitimate resource, is the ultimate consequence of this structure.

Chapter 9 examines generational changes among femicide perpetrators in the region. This chapter investigates variations in "narrative voice" that reflect the historical moment we are navigating. Comparing the stories of men born in the 1950s and 1960s—who experienced the early stirrings of organised women's rights movements, alongside parallel dictatorships and patriarchal backlash—with those of men born in the 1990s and early 2000s—when feminist ideas and human rights logic had gradually been incorporated into states and daily life, albeit not without resistance—reveals this transformation. While core narrative elements have remained consistent, younger perpetrators told stories with a reduced sense of impunity, less implicit social support, diminished victim-blaming, and a decline in the bravado with which aggression is described.

Chapter 10 presents an ad hoc breaching experiment: non-violence specialised scholars were given altered vignettes from this book—some with gender-swapped characters, others replacing femicide with a non-physically aggressive conflict. Responses varied between experiencing narrative dissonance (expressed as 'What?!' reactions) and finding plausibility alignment ('I get it' responses). Both interpretations highlight the persistence of gender scripts—and the ways in which they are justified. Aiming to engage readers ('us') and offer a closer look at how narratives circulate beyond perpetrators, the chapter demonstrates just how dominant these narratives are. It also focuses on the epistemological problem of othering violence and excluding ourselves from the equation. Ultimately, in this chapter I advocate for a more inclusive understanding of the narratives that foster violence—presenting this as a way to counteract penal spectatorship.

Finally, Chapter 11 concludes the book by addressing four key aspects. It explores how focusing on stories requires valuing language as both a source and a medium through which patriarchal norms and gender structures are enacted. It then revisits the book's main empirical discussions, synthesising key findings. Attention is also given to the spaces where these narratives are most intensely reproduced, highlighting critical junctures that could serve as potential intervention points. The book closes with a reflection on the current state of policy interventions, considering their limitations and future directions.

That said, I would like to point out that the book adopts a hybrid genre, drawing from two distinct writing traditions. Firstly, this work is heavily inspired by Messerschmidt's *Nine Lives* (2000). The structure of this seminal text is particularly useful for illustrating the interconnections among biographies, narratives, and violence. This should be evident in Parts II and III. Secondly, I have chosen to present the vignettes in a more literary style, as fiction often engages a wider audience. This approach draws on elements from the tradition of investigative journalism in Latin America, which frequently intersects with anthropological work. As Carrión (2018) describes, this genre—commonly referred to as the *chronicle*—"is a journalistic form that allows for the exploration of emotional worlds, the colours of landscapes, and the nuances of language with greater freedom" (my translation) (p. 10).

A final note: At the beginning of each vignette, you will find an illustration. Like the cover art, these images are not intended to evoke repulsion or portray the interviewed men as monsters. Instead, they are meant to ground a deeply material topic and provide a brief escape from written narration. I believe that images are both mnemonic and heuristic tools, offering another powerful way to convey meaning.

2

Why?

Broader Context

> The crisis consists precisely in the fact that the old is dying and the new cannot be born; in this interregnum a great variety of morbid symptoms appear. (Gramsci, 1971 [1929–1935], p. 276)

Femicide is broadly defined as the killing of women and girls due to their gender. Coined by Diana Russell in 1976, the term encompasses murders that are profoundly shaped by gendered power dynamics, such as honour killings, murders following rape, and lethal violence after prolonged abusive relationships. In feminist literature, femicide and feminicide are frequently differentiated, with femicide typically used to highlight individual acts of violence, while feminicide is understood to focus on structural phenomena—a term that emphasises the systemic nature of the issue and the complicity of state institutions in its perpetuation (Lagarde, 2006). While this distinction may have been useful in the early development of the field—when critical analytical frameworks were being established—today we can recognise both terms as equally pointing to the structural nature of these killings and the various forms

M. H. Di Marco, *Narratives of Femicide Perpetrators in Latin America*,
https://doi.org/10.1007/978-3-031-97367-3_2

of collective complicity. This book explores intimate femicide—homicides committed by partners or ex-partners—through the lens of the perpetrators' narratives.

The term femicide foregrounds not only an extreme form of male-chauvinist violence but also its disproportionate nature. Women are killed by partners, ex-partners, and family members at significantly higher rates than men (UNODC & UN Women, 2024). They are six times more likely than men to be killed by someone with whom they share a close relationship. This persistent trend is evident across most countries and sustained over decades, reinforcing the claim that femicide is a global problem.

However, the global criminological landscape regarding femicide is far from uniform. The latest United Nations Office on Drugs and Crime (UNODC) report (2024) reveals a complex picture. For instance, Europe recorded a 21% decline in female intimate partner and family-related homicides between 2010 and 2022, while the Americas experienced an increase over the same period. Sub-regional and national variations paint a nuanced picture that defies simple explanations. For instance, between 2017 and 2022 (the period for which data is accessible for comparison), femicide rates fell in Central and South America, whereas North America and the Caribbean saw increases. In the United States, for instance, there was a notable spike during the COVID-19 pandemic.

This statistical landscape presents a paradox. While global homicide rates have generally declined—likely due to demographic changes and criminological transitions (Pridemore, 2007)—femicide rates in some regions remain stable or are rising, like Latin America. Verkko's Laws (1951) have been fairly robust in explaining that these fluctuations in homicide rates are primarily driven by variations in male-on-male homicides. Verkko observed that in societies with high overall homicide rates, most victims tend to be men, primarily due to male-on-male violence. However, as overall homicide rates decline, the proportion of female victims tends to increase, not necessarily because femicides rise, but because male-on-male homicides decrease more sharply.

Still, understanding this phenomenon has sparked broader debates. Why is this form of violence more prevalent in certain places than others? For instance, backlash theories suggest that femicide rates may rise as reactionary forces push back against gender equality. This issue becomes even more complex when considering well-founded criticisms regarding reporting issues, under-registration, different data sources, and the varying operationalisations of femicide across different countries, all of which may distort a global statistical reading of femicide.

In Latin America, femicide looms over society like the sword of Damocles, shaping not only the lives of women and girls but also broader socio-political realities. The term itself has gained widespread traction, embraced by social movements, popular feminism, and, more recently, even by state-led initiatives. These efforts have fostered diverse programmes, identities, and discourses addressing the issue. Notable examples include the *Ni Una Menos* movement across the region, alliances with Indigenous activism in Peru, discussions surrounding the murders in Ciudad Juárez in Mexico, and debates about Brazil's Maria da Penha Femicide law. Together, these examples illustrate the evolving landscape of femicide's conceptualisation and its multifaceted usage across the region.

Impunity—a word that has become both a political focal point and an analytical framework—has made femicide a particularly significant political term in Latin America. For decades, even in ostensibly modern legal systems, the killing of women was often misclassified as suicides or accidents, dismissed as unrelated to gender-based violence or, at best, categorised as crimes of passion (Fernández, 2012; Ruggiero, 2001). Institutional barriers and inadequate training of key actors exacerbated this issue (Alvelais et al., 2019). These misclassifications detached femicide from broader gender structures, allowing impunity to persist through discourses and practices that obscured the operation of patriarchy. Even after femicide-specific laws were enacted, impunity persists due to the lack of effective prosecution or even the failure to allocate resources to address the issue (Brunke & Boira, 2021).

While the killing of women due to their gender is not confined to any specific region, debates and political organisation around femicide have largely remained regional. Despite its prominence in Latin America, the term remains largely unused in the Global North and other parts of the world. As a result, protocols, media portrayals, and institutional responses in Latin America have acquired distinctive features, marked by greater visibility and organisation.

Worldwide, however, public discourse on intimate partner homicide has undergone significant changes over the past two decades. Awareness of violence against women and the political will to address it have grown globally, permeating institutions, media, and popular culture. Social movements and institutional initiatives have been pivotal in making these concerns visible, creating networks within both state and international structures. Moreover, a series of international developments have shaped the advocacy, research, and policy landscape surrounding femicide. Statistical recording and the standardisation of measurements, such as the *Statistical Framework for Measuring the Gender-Related Killing of Women and Girls* (UNWomen & UNODC, 2022), have become central strategies for addressing the issue. Continuous surveillance and regular reporting by organisations like the UNODC, alongside national femicide registries and media monitors, have significantly contributed to recognising femicide as a social issue. This aligns with what Gusfield (1984) coined as the "construction of a public problem".

These transformations have not been without controversy. Critics argue that the co-option of femicide by state and international agendas has diluted critical discussions, such as those addressing state responsibility (Cole & Phillips, 2008; Segato, 2016; Whynacht, 2019). Others highlight limitations in current measurement practices (Walklate & Fitz-Gibbon, 2023), the politics of data concealment and selection (Kohan, 2021; Posey, 2023), and questions about who collects data and how (D'Ignazio, 2024; Suárez Val et al., 2023). The lack of reliable data and the overemphasis on risk factor analyses (Gnisci & Pace, 2016), along with debates on the definitional contours and context-specific applicability of the term (Viveros-Vigoya, 2016), underscore the complexity of femicide.

These debates partly reflect the emergence and current state of the field. The tensions surrounding the definition of femicide, as well as the challenges in determining how to study and prevent it, are perhaps inherent to the process itself. However, they also highlight the growing recognition of femicide's multifaceted nature. Within these discussions, the limited attention given to understanding perpetration itself highlights a crucial yet often-overlooked aspect: the men who commit femicide.

In this context, I argue that alternative methods that incorporate the subjective underpinnings of this phenomenon are crucial for untangling its persistence. Examining the stories of those who commit violence—indeed, a tricky endeavour—provides a valuable lens for understanding how meaning is constructed within their rationalities and how culture becomes mechanised. These stories are also a gateway to decode the regular patterns of femicide in the region.

Purpose and Argument

In *Decline of the English Murder*, George Orwell (1978 [1946]) famously sketches the profile of what he considers to be the most typical murderer. Ideally, this man would be a solicitor or a doctor, perhaps a respectable politician or a staunch advocate against alcohol. While his crime might appear to arise from feelings of passion for his secretary, his true motive would be the fear of public humiliation. Poisoning his wife seems a far less scandalous option than enduring the disgrace of a divorce (Worsley, 2014, p. 1). Orwell entertains us by playing with our assumptions about the emotions driving these men to murder, yet he does so with irony. After all, our preconceptions often bear little relation to the actual workings of their minds.

This book flips the conventional script and asks instead: what do the stories of men who have killed their partners and ex-partners reveal about their relationships and worldviews? Are there recurring patterns of interpretation across Latin America? By examining the stories these men construct, I explore how patriarchal structures are enacted in concrete cases of intimate femicides. In doing so, I identify common narrative patterns linked to femicides across Latin American countries, while also exploring generational differences in the stories men tell.

Scholars such as Presser (2013) and Smith (2005) have argued that uncovering the link between specific stories and the actions they prompt can provide a productive lens through which to understand social phenomena. In exploring the stories of perpetrators, I aim to shift the conversation away from expert knowledge that tends to, on the one hand, either individualise and decontextualise violence, or, on the other hand, reduce these actors to overly deterministic or fatalistic views—treating them as mere automata of patriarchy. Instead, I seek to foster a discussion that acknowledges the creative nature of social action.

The two approaches ultimately aim to strike a balance between individuality and determinism. Avoiding individualisation should, after so many decades of feminist mobilisation, come as no surprise. Violence against women does not operate in isolation, but is embedded in our societies. The argument that femicide is a product of our societies is not new, but it still faces resistance. The other argument, however, is somewhat more novel: going beyond a superficial structuralist analysis of femicide as a purely cultural product, where perpetrators are treated as mere cultural dupes (Garfinkel, 1967). Like culture, patriarchy is a vast concept that resists simple applications. Abstract theorisation about gender-based violence may be necessary to understand its contours, but it can also leave little room for complexity.

This work aims to break down and make manageable broader concepts including femicide and machismo, which have been central to many contemporary discussions. While these discussions are valuable, they inevitably raise new problematic issues. The one I address here is the banalisation of the rationality of perpetrators. This oversimplification can take various forms, whether in the language of risk factors, psychologising labels, or in portrayals of perpetrators as outlier evil doers or as 'sons of patriarchy'. This is not intended as a critique of feminism per se, but rather as an expansion of the current discussion, offering an opportunity to provide empirically grounded arguments.

There are numerous ways to unpacked 'femicide culture' into more operational concepts. My approach examines narratives of femicide as socially constructs that are embodied by real individuals navigating their everyday thoughts and emotions. I will often emphasise that these narratives are deeply embedded in power dynamics—shaped by choices, constraints, and controls. Some are marked by intense emotion, while others remain shrouded in painful silence.

Ken Plummer (1995, p. 16) persuasively insisted that stories "make a difference". They are more than mere words or discourses; they represent the organisation of knowledge, the communication of ideas, and the embodiment of social scripts. In his words, "society itself may be seen as a textured but seamless web of stories emerging everywhere through interaction: holding people together, pulling people apart, making societies work" (p. 7). Narratives can instigate or mitigate wars (Smith, 2005), shape the reconstruction of past experiences (Rosenthal, 2010), challenge dominant societal norms (Halberstam, 2011), influence our experiences of illness (Sontag, 2003), and even inform who is included and excluded from history (Alexievich, 2017). Through these various roles, narratives not only shape personal identities and collective memory but also construct the very foundations of societal power structures.

The focus on perpetrators' stories in this book is grounded on three premises. The first is that understanding femicide requires careful consideration of the act itself. This premise challenges the tendency to place the responsibility for preventing femicide solely on women and legal frameworks. As such, this book intends to contribute to the ongoing shift towards examining masculinities. The second premise acknowledges that, despite the need to understand these men, there remains a significant lack of research on their lives and perspectives. Finally, this lacuna has inevitably hindered the development of theories concerning femicide perpetration. As Segato (2003) has long argued, we end up knowing about the contours of gender-based violence, but not the rationality underpinning it.

This book's narrative approach leads us to four key arguments. First, widespread and shared narratives surrounding women, relationships, jealousy, and possessiveness shape lethal violence. The common thread is that violence is used instrumentally to punish and uphold a moral norm, with the disruption of an expectation serving as a key turning point. Second, femicide narratives are supported by broader stories about social relationships, particularly those involving male peers and toothless institutional responses that ultimately endorse violence and impunity. Without these surrounding stories, femicide is difficult to fully comprehend. This argument, which has been less visible in current discussions, highlights the persistent legitimacy of intimate partner violence within social and institutional contexts. Third, even in extreme cases where language is disorganised or individuals express no remorse, narrative structures remain, influencing how perpetrators make sense of their crimes and reflecting ingrained misogyny. Cases that might be readily pathologised can also be still understood through a sociological framework. Finally, when examining narratives across generations, there is a noticeable decline in impunity, victim-blaming, and bravado ingrained in the stories. Younger men increasingly rely on justifications and excuses—indirectly altering the narratives—reflecting a broader historical shift shaped by feminist movements and human rights discourses.

At its core, this argument addresses the legitimacy of femicide in our language, illustrating how circulating stories inscribe the possibility of such violence. Furthermore, this book argues that a reliance on friendships, institutions, and individuals to support violence or, at the very least, fail to intervene, plays a crucial role in these crimes. Collectively, these elements form a master narrative.

I invite the reader to subscribe, if only momentarily, to this theoretical framework. To embrace the potential of narratives and avoid ready-made labels is to delve deeper into this issue. By providing detailed accounts, I seek to upend clichéd, formulaic ideas about intimate partner violence. The book is rich in anecdotes, experiences, paradoxes, and ambiguities—all of which are part of the reality of people's stories.

The book is written with the hope of providing more tools to understand this form of harm and, hopefully, inspire efforts for prevention. I aim to repoliticise these narratives as a façade of patriarchy. My assumption is that othering perpetrators as 'black sheep' causes more harm than good in our current context. By excluding ourselves from the group of misogynists, we create an epistemological problem, presuming they possess something we do not. Is this true? By bracketing our assumptions about murder and violence as an analytical strategy, we can learn a great deal about. As Renahan notes in the context of domestic violence perpetrator programmes, it is essential to "humanise the traumatising but traumatised men" with whom we interact (2021, p. 324).

Academic Trends

This book was not written in isolation; it emerged, as previously argued, within a specific context where femicide—as an analytical term, a political movement, and an empirical reality—continues to evolve. Since the 1990s, the literature on femicide has expanded across disciplines, establishing itself as a recognised field. Crucially, this body of work has not been limited to a single perspective. Recent compendiums, such as Dawson & Mobayed (2023) or Devaney et al. (2021), highlight dominant foci in the field: risk factors, risk assessment tools, policing responses and penal codes, the standardisation of measurement, fatality reviews, and analyses of rates and macro-social trends. Longstanding scholarship on patriarchal social conditions that enable femicide remains central. Less prominently, studies have explored prevention strategies, the roles of families and kinship networks, the advocacy of social movements for justice, and the impact on survivors and communities. These diverse approaches underscore the multifaceted nature of femicide as a subject of inquiry.

Mainstream academic discussions of perpetrators, however, remain less prominent. A quick search of any major research database reveals that most studies on this topic either employ quantitative methods to identify risk factors (e.g., age, employment status) or focus on the mental health or behaviours of offenders (e.g., psychopathologies, coercive control strategies). Most strikingly, much of this research relies on secondary sources that, to varying degrees, only address perpetrators indirectly. These approaches have undoubtedly provided a crucial foundation for the field and, more importantly, have informed the development of strategies to intervene and prevent the killing of women.

Browsing the internet once again, one might encounter sweeping statements such as: 'Most homicide perpetrators are unemployed and have a history of substance abuse', 'Femicide is the result of deeply misogynistic men', or 'She was dealing with a real monster'. Less rigorous sources might attribute the murder to events happening 'out of the blue', alcohol or drug use, or even the woman's own actions. When exploring risk factors for intimate femicide, I was particularly struck by findings that highlight certain markers of heightened risk: a history of intimate partner violence, non-lethal strangulation, and extreme jealousy or controlling behaviours, such as isolating the victim or monitoring her activities.

This situation has led to a current impasse: while there is growing interest in this phenomenon, accompanied by greater resources and prevention efforts, the rationality of those who commit femicide is often overlooked. For instance, a recent systematic review identified only 14 studies that delve into the lives and perspectives of these individuals using first-hand qualitative information (Evans et al., 2023). Ultimately, femicide perpetrators are heavily discussed and referenced by others, but we rarely hear from them in their own words.

A longstanding critique has centred on the usefulness of understanding people's rationality, or as Oddone (2017) eloquently states, the need to 'focus' on the men. While this critique has come in many shades, it always downplays the importance of subjectivity and agency, sometimes reducing people to 'Cartesian automata'. One way in which this type of reductionism has operated is with the reification of the risk factor approach (e.g., Douglas, 1997; Farmer, 2009; Menéndez, 2008; Scheper-Hughes, 1997), which treats complex social issues as isolated, measurable variables, ignoring the broader, interconnected contexts that shape individual actions.

In essence, the question of subjectivity I pose here is: how do these factors operate? What does jealousy and control mean for aggressors? Are there underpinning narratives that shed light on the logic of violence? This inquiry seeks to understand how these aspects are not merely triggers but part of a broader narrative shaped by societal contexts, offering deeper insights into the motivations and rationalities behind acts of violence.

A Shift Towards Perpetrators

> In general it must be said: people whose business it is to attend trials, court reporters by profession or by chance like me, are more fascinated by the culprits than by their victims. We feel sorry for the victims, but

> it's the culprits whose personalities we try to understand. It's their lives we scrutinise in search of the snag, the mysterious point at which they veered towards lying or crime. (Carrère, 2024, p. 113)

Scholarly interest in offenders' biographies and logics is far from new. Much like Emmanuel Carrère's logic in his chronicle of the terrorist attacks in France, the interest in understanding those who harm is fuelled by the complexity of inflicting harm. Classical works in the social sciences—dating back to the Chicago School—have laid the groundwork for nearly a century of research on the subject. However, the scholarship on intimate partner violence offenders in general is fairly recent and, when it comes to femicide specifically, remains scarce.

At its core, there are two main themes that can be explored when examining perpetrators. One concerns their trajectories. Much of the discussion has focused on identifying moments in their lives that might provide clues to their later abusive behaviour. Some studies have examined prior violence-related criminal records (e.g., Dobash & Dobash, 2017) and the extent to which physical violence precedes intimate femicide (Johnson et al., 2019). Others have explored femicide pathways and their social contexts (Goussinsky & Yassour-Borochowitz, 2012), as well as adverse childhood experiences and their impact on emotional vulnerability (Mathews et al., 2011).

The perspectives of these men have also been explored. The focus has been on understanding how they rationalise homicide—for instance, through neutralisation strategies and moral disengagement (Di Marco & Evans, 2020; Regis-Moura et al., 2021). While varied, most of this research has highlighted, in different ways, the emotional dimensions associated with homicide. A striking similarity across much of the research is the sense of deep despair that compels these men to act, irrespective of the consequences (Goussinsky & Yassour-Borochowitz, 2012). Male-chauvinist narratives frequently evoke feelings of anger and a sense of being 'out of control', as well as profound emotional turmoil and vulnerability (Mathews et al., 2015), including the fear of losing a partner as a key emotional trigger.

Ultimately, most discussions that feature the perspectives of perpetrators suggest that violence is often seen as a means to address perceived emotional damage (Fahs et al., 2023). Aggrieved entitlement, for instance, can offer a way to decode how normalised experiences within a system come into crisis when challenged (Kimmel, 2019). This subjective position appears logical when we consider that the hallmarks of hegemonic masculinity include aggression, a lack of emotional acknowledgement, and the rejection of any association with femininity (Berggren et al., 2021; Connell & Messerschmidt, 2005).

When considering the systemic nature of violence in Latin America, it makes sense that some, like Segato (2016, 2024), argue femicide is not merely an act of violence. For perpetrators, femicide is often framed as a response to perceived challenges to their selft or sense of control, but it also functions as a form of communication. It reminds women of their subordinate roles and sends a message to other men that masculine dominance must be enforced. This interpretation underscores the discourses that shape perpetrators' actions, where violence becomes a tool to reassert authority and uphold gender hierarchies.

Despite a growing interest in this topic, it remains a marginal endeavour when compared to the substantial attention given to other aspects of violence. This is particularly significant, as we cannot equate perpetrators of intimate partner violence and femicide. My main concern, however, is that most broad discussions on femicide still resort to the 'bad apple' approach or 'drown' perpetrators in structural explanations, eliminating any nuances. The lack of interest in an agentic interpretation of perpetration means we are left without the necessary tools to understand why these acts occur.

I advocate for a more politically savvy approach in how we compartmentalise research in this field. The policing of disciplinary boundaries—separating agency from structure, subject from context, etc.—has real consequences for knowledge production. Yet, it is by bridging these epistemologies and interests that we can create better opportunities for explaining and ultimately preventing femicides.

About the Labels

A final issue concerns the language used, as words ultimately lie at the heart of this book. The disciplinary diversity of the field is evident in the terminology employed. Terms such as 'offenders', 'perpetrators', 'killers', 'murderers', 'harm-doers', 'harm-users', 'aggressors', and 'abusers' form a broad lexicon for describing these men. Yet, these terms are far from neutral. Is it the same to refer to someone as a homicide offender or as a murderer? Can an individual who committed femicide be used interchangeably with these other labels?

The way these men are categorised reflects both a theoretical choice and a political stance on violence. Consider the difference between describing someone as a violent man, implying a constant attribute, versus a man who used violence, which foregrounds the action itself. Terminology, as a discursive contract (Foucault, 2002), has real consequences for where we direct our attention and focus.

Still, this discussion goes beyond terminology alone. The terms we use to describe violent acts are tied to the systems of knowledge that produce them (Bruner, 2002). Labels like 'violent man', 'homicidal pact', 'premeditation', and 'intent' shape how we view violence, turning it into something we can analyse and categorise. The different terms used by the media, courts, mental health institutions, prisons, and those used in common parlance not only reveal competing ideas but also reflect the different ways each group views violence. These terms shape our understanding of violence by guiding our focus towards certain elements and away from others. Without questioning them, we limit our ability to fully grasp the complexities behind violent acts. Choosing one term over another can obscure deeper issues, such as the potential for change, either on an individual level or within broader societal shifts.

This discussion has also prompted Robben and Laban Hinton (2023) to argue that "perpetrator studies too often get stuck in static typologies due to the figurations that inform the field" (p. 14). One such figuration contrasts the perpetrator as a monster with the notion of an ordinary human being. The fact that much of perpetrator research still rests on assumptions of innate, constant features, or Cartesian rationality, signals a need for more nuanced discussions.

In this book, I use the term perpetrator (*perpetrador* in Spanish, the primary language of my fieldwork) to emphasise the act itself and foreground the performance of violence, acknowledging that this label does not capture any essential aspect of the individuals in question. I argue that we must move away from essentialist views of violence (Moriconi Bezerra, 2013) and static representations of femicide that equate individuals with the violence they commit. With this, I aim to strike a balance between approaches—one where we acknowledge the harm done, and one that also considers, in line with the idea of the banality of evil (Arendt, 2006 [1963]), how perpetrators, often ordinary individuals, are shaped by social structures, norms, and processes that enable violence. This perspective allows for a more complex understanding of this crime, one that recognises the interplay between individual agency and the broader societal forces that influence violent behaviour.

3
What?

A Narrative World

> The limits of my language mean the limits of my world. (Wittgestein, 2021 [1921], p. 74).

This book is fundamentally about the stories people tell. By stories, I do not mean anything obscure or convoluted, but rather the straightforward tales individuals share to convey meaning. In conversations with these men, they employed a narrative arc to illustrate a point: they began by setting the scene with initial details, described the central 'knot' of what transpired, and then brought the story to a conclusion. They might have recounted a story to reconstruct a period of their life or simply to express a feeling they experienced on a particular day. In every case, these narrative arcs are the focus of this inquiry.

Opting to explore the stories of femicide perpetrators is far from superfluous. Jerome Bruner (2002) famously discussed the 'tyranny of the narrative', arguing that while our reality is not entirely narrative—an idea supported by discourse theorists ranging from Bakhtin and Todorov to Foucault—narratives are inextricably linked to real-world

M. H. Di Marco, *Narratives of Femicide Perpetrators in Latin America*,
https://doi.org/10.1007/978-3-031-97367-3_3

events. Meaning is not solely denotative; it also encompasses connotations, emotions, and cultural implications that extend beyond the literal definition. Meaning operates within language and cultural communication, not only representing but also subjectively implying and guiding actions. Ultimately, this implies that we cannot think beyond narrative frameworks: nothing is accessible or comprehensible outside the boundaries of our narratives.

From this perspective, there is no such thing as an unspeakable truth. In my view of language, if meanings exist, there are words to express them. Similarly, if there is discourse, there are signifiers. This idea forms a central premise of this book, as violence is often depicted as an irrational and inexpressible phenomenon. The portrayal of femicides as 'inexplicable actions', 'out of the blue killings', or based on 'unexpected behaviour' not only obscures the broader patterns in which femicides occur but also tends to obscure the social conditions that enable them. In reality, nothing is more describable or addressable than violence, particularly when various discourses on violence (Binik, 2020) attempt to decipher its logic.

Language and Recipes

This book aims to uncover patterns in the ways perpetrators narrate their experiences of femicide, seeking to link these individual accounts to a broader, shared rationality across Latin America. The key is to understand the function of these stories within their social contexts. Are these men merely reconstructing events, or are their stories shaped by dominant master narratives? Or perhaps are they entirely tailored to the audience? These are the questions that, in one way or another, lie at the heart of all scholarship on aggressors, from genocide perpetrators (Feld & Salvi, 2019; Robben, 2014) to batterers (Hearn, 1998).

A starting point is that we are, indeed, expert storytellers (Ricœur, 2004). The daily use of stories is an unavoidable aspect of life: we weave narratives not only in our everyday interactions but also as a fundamental means of navigating existence. Whether at school, work, or on a date, we are constantly constructing and reshaping stories to suit the context and the perceived arc of our lives. We also rely on narratives when making decisions about our actions. With stories, we indeed "transfigure the banal" (Danto, 1994), imbuing everyday experiences with deeper significance. However, we often lack awareness of how profoundly narratives shape our reality.

Understanding stories can be a complex endeavour. Since we have inevitably naturalised them, narratives often appear elusive and layered—what Bruner (1990) described as "nebulous". We rarely pause to acknowledge or reflect on the stories we have absorbed about love, friendship, or frustration. Yet, precisely because of their frequently unquestioned nature, narratives serve as powerful vehicles for social norms, shaping how we interpret and recount human experiences. Having heard them endlessly throughout our lives, their unexamined presence profoundly influences us. This underscores the enduring challenge of interpreting our own practices while remaining embedded within the same social systems—a dynamic encapsulated in the double hermeneutics (Giddens, 1984) where any critical examination of society is shaped by the very norms we seek to analyse.

A key principle here is that narratives are the byproduct of our relationships. This principle is central to a microsociological understanding of language (Gergen, 1991): while we are exposed to narratives, we incorporate them in specific ways, make them our own, and enact them situationally. This process underpins not only the social construction of reality—acknowledging both a preexisting reality shaped by past interactions and one actively put into motion in the present—but also the idea that there is an interaction between individuals taking place in the core of society.

The issue that becomes relevant now is one of learning and socialisation: ultimately, how do these narratives become part of our repertoire for understanding others and acting in the world? A classic approach to answering this question is through the concept of language games (Winch, 2018; Wittgenstein, 2009 [1953]): the idea that meaning emerges from use within specific social contexts. Children—and adults—often learn these games through practice rather than explicit instruction. Similarly, we acquire narratives through practical engagement rather than formal understanding. We are exposed to them when watching television, reading books, or gossiping with our neighbours. Just as children grasp the intricacies of a game through play and interaction with peers, individuals come to understand language and social narratives through lived experiences and participation in their communities. This highlights a fundamental asymmetry between doing and understanding, akin to learning a new card game: while you could read the rules, true comprehension often comes from simply playing.

The metaphor of a recipe effectively illustrates this idea, offering an analogy that has been valuable both for this book and for my own understanding. We can follow a recipe as written, but we can also alter, adapt, and transform it. Often, we learn recipes by watching our relatives and friends prepare meals. Similarly, gender narratives are embedded in cultural products—books, laws, fashion. We see others following these narratives, telling particular stories, and upholding specific values. While we recognise their presence and the influence they exert, we also hold the power to challenge and reshape them.

Understanding narratives in this way makes it clear that storytelling is not merely a way of interpreting reality but also of constructing ourselves and the social structures around us. Individuals might adjust these narratives, alter the ingredients, and achieve different outcomes, but ultimately, we rely on these 'recipes' as templates for action. In this sense, these recipes are neither teleological nor deterministic; they do not exert absolute control over us. There is no overarching structure governing our behaviour without our active participation. We create society—its institutions, norms, harms, and protections—through our daily interpretations and reinterpretations of these narratives. Ultimately, the everyday, taken-for-granted actions and interactions through which people make sense of their lives are also the means by which they shape and uphold society (Garfinkel, 1967). Meaning arises through these stories, but this is not an external force that constrains us. Rather, it is something we have internalised, even embodied, and put into practice.

It becomes clear that storytelling itself is a social action, an integral part of maintaining social structures (such as patriarchy). The focus here, therefore, is on how these stories foster action. Just like stories about love shape our expectations of relationships, cultural scripts that romanticise jealousy as proof of love (Illouz, 2013) can legitimise control, paving the way for violence. Regardless of the specific terms used to describe these stories—scripts, narrative structures, recipes, schemas—this approach underscores that structure and action coexist and shape one another. Social systems, after all, are the products of individual actions.

Finally, I find it useful to make explicit the temporality of this connection. As Presser and Sandberg (2015) argue, narratives can be treated as an "independent variable": narratives predate individuals and may be seen as conditioning factors, albeit through the interpretative work of those individuals. This implies two points for the analytical task of decoding these femicide stories: first, that narratives exist prior to action; and second, that the availability of these narratives can act as an instigator for action. It is important to note that causality is not part of this epistemological framework—not because it is dismissed, but because it is incongruent with this hermeneutic understanding of social reality.

Viewing narratives *as conditions that set the stage for* action can help connect men's life stories to their social context and, ultimately, to the broader issue of violence against women as a societal problem. These stories, while told by individual men, are not entirely original creations. They may contain ad hoc components shaped by social contexts and individual circumstances, but they are drawn from a broader repertoire of available narratives. The key point is that these dominant narratives deserve our focus precisely because they are being used. This also shows that narratives are both normative and are, in fact, part of our daily actions—from thinking and imagining to acting on ideas.

Understanding Recipes

The aim thus far has been to refine our understanding of narratives and their significance. This naturally raises the questions: Are we seeking to understand motivations, or are we examining the collective conditions that shape them? And what value do these stories hold? In response, I focus on three central ideas: motivation, context, and veracity.

People craft and share stories about their past actions, drawing on various "vocabularies of motive" to articulate their reasons (Wright Mills, 1940). These motivational stories are inevitably framed within a discursive context: what is told is shaped not only by the social environment but also by the present moment (Berger & Luckmann, 2017 [1966]). This leads us to ask: what exactly are the interviewed men revealing in their stories?

A common approach involves seeking subjective meanings that directly link action to intention (e.g., 'I did X because of Y in context Z'). This method typically establishes a causal relationship between an action and its stated motivation, assuming that the accounts provided by perpetrators offer direct access to their past motivations—as if the definitive clue to understanding femicides lies hidden within their stories. The issue with this perspective is that it presumes a fixed, consciously acknowledged reason for an action, one that remains constant over time. By this logic, shifts in social discourse would have little influence on how motivations are narrated. For example, we might analyse in the present an interview with a man who described his partner in overtly misogynistic terms during the late 1980s, without fully accounting for how the cultural climate of that period shaped his narrative. This approach fails to account for discursive frameworks—such as judicial or psychological ones—that shape how individuals connect past events to their 'inner motivations' (Bruner, 2002).

Instead, people's stories can be understood as drawing upon their available stock of knowledge (Schutz, 1967). For the men interviewed, this stock of knowledge might include discourses on normativity, entitlement, and domination, as well as narratives surrounding family formation, fidelity, and legitimate violence. Viewing stories through this lens avoids the pitfalls of causally linking motivations to actions (Gergen, 1994) and instead highlights the role of dominant discourses in shaping these narratives.

This book is dedicated to exploring how the stories told by these men provide insights into broader narratives at play. These insights are made apparent in the selection and thematisation that occur during biographical work (Riemann, 2006). Interviewees identify elements they perceive as central to their life stories, emphasising specific themes that come to define their narratives. This selection process is shaped not only by how individuals wish to be perceived but also by their interpretation of certain memories' significance and what is ultimately deemed legitimate to share. It underscores that any reconstruction of lived experience is inherently incomplete, influenced by subjective interpretation rather than being a purely factual recounting.

This argument should make evident that shifting contexts impact storytelling. Different contexts offer distinct resources for storytelling, as each setting fosters, restricts, and shapes the narrative process in unique ways. Historical conditions, for instance, may lead men to justify physical abuse through victim-blaming or by citing a temporary loss of control. In other cases, humour may serve as a means of rationalising violence (Stanko & Hobdell, 1993). More overtly, allegations of witchcraft or claims that a woman violated honour codes have been used as defences for homicide, proving effective in certain cultural contexts (Adinkrah, 2004; Husseini, 2009).

This brings us to the question of veracity. Researchers often aim to separate fact from fiction. Yet in this line of fieldwork, this dichotomy frequently proves inadequate—hence the emergence of the "fiction-reality continuum" to reframe this discussion (Plummer, 2019). Even honest informants may misremember events, and many narratives, in turn, resist simple fact-checking. Beliefs and myths, for example, cannot be weighed against other 'facts' in the usual sense. Similarly, the value of narratives about violence—what individuals witnessed, did, felt, or heard—may rest less on their 'accuracy' and more on the meaning narrators assign to violent events.

When speaking with perpetrators, these fictions may prove more insightful than life-course facts. Rumours, fabrications, denials, evasions, and silences—what Fuji (2010) calls "meta-data" in interviews—can reveal norms that influence femicide itself. These elements are integral to the data in this book, as they show how present-day conditions shape what people are willing to disclose about past violence, as well as what they might choose to embellish, minimise, or withhold.

Ultimately, the book's primary focus is on the stories themselves. Veracity, completeness, coherence, and testability are secondary concerns. Instead, the emphasis lies on patterns of storytelling. The accounts of different men across the region, detailing their lives and the crimes they committed, contribute to a collective stock of knowledge that warrants in-depth exploration.

Not Just a Story, Not Just Fate

> Emotions are not just something 'we have' but are also ways of being involved in the world. They shape the surface of bodies and worlds, creating the very impressions that we have of ourselves and others. (Ahmed, 2004, p. 4)

Stories are neither loose nor innocuous constructs; they are not simply products of individual consciousness, nor are they entirely shaped by personal will or imposed from above. Despite their ideal nature (or even superstructural one), stories exert tangible effects on the material world: they shape how people act, feel, and perceive their place in society, as Ahmed (2004) vividly argues. We marry, build careers, vote, and even recycle in alignment with particular narratives. Conversely, we may feel devalued or displaced when these narratives challenge our bodies, sexualities, or identities—all in response to the stories we inhabit.

This chapter began with a reference to the "tyranny of the narrative", aiming to highlight how the persistence of intimate femicides in Latin America can be understood from a cultural perspective that is often overlooked, oversimplified, or disregarded. However, this should not lead to the false impression that change is unattainable. The fact that we cannot exist outside of language speaks to the essence of the human condition (Lacan, 1973), but this is not meant in a purely constraining sense. Language can also be subversive, as it provides the means through which power structures can be questioned and reconfigured (Butler, 2006). The mere existence of the words femicide and feminicide could be seen as the result of such processes. Change occurs through discursive transformation, whether it involves an individual shift in identity or desistance, or the emergence of a social movement that fosters collective change. In either case, the pathway to change passes through discourse.

Acknowledging this potential for change is not only meant to reassure but also serves as a guiding principle for our work. The following chapters delve into the reasoning behind violent misogynistic crimes, with the aim of grasping more than just the specifics of each individual case. It would be shortsighted to explore this topic without considering its dynamic nature over time, as is further explored in Chapter 9. Change should be part of our focus, as well as the patterns sustaining these crimes.

The study of narratives that foster femicide not only reveals their persistence in Latin America but also presents a powerful avenue for contemplating intervention and collective responsibility. Notably, "lived experiences with *causing harm* can be an asset to our [feminist] movement" (emphasis in the original) (Whynacht, 2019, p. 26). Only by studying these stories can we gain a deeper understanding of the social frameworks at play, and how to reshape them.

4
How?

This chapter delves 'behind the curtain of the research' and describes the trajectory that lead to this book: not only the procedures I followed to examine narratives about femicide but also the decisions that gave this research its specific features. Given the complexities of working on violence, and especially with perpetrators in Latin American prisons, uncovering what Becker (1998) called the *how*—including the detours, dead ends, and unexpected turns of fieldwork—is as much a reflection of the subject matter as the words of the men themselves.

Fieldwork

This research draws on fieldwork conducted in medium- and maximum-security prisons across seven countries in Latin America over eight years (2016–2023): Argentina, Bolivia, Chile, Honduras, Mexico, Paraguay, and Venezuela. The interviews were primarily conducted by me, though some were carried out by colleagues pursuing their own research or by research assistants involved in the Crime in Latin America (CRIMLA)

M. H. Di Marco, *Narratives of Femicide Perpetrators in Latin America*, https://doi.org/10.1007/978-3-031-97367-3_4

project which aimed to develop a theoretically grounded, culturally, and contextually sensitive life-course criminology of Latin America.[1]

Gaining access to the prisons was the first and most time-consuming stage of fieldwork. Given the project's framework and the structure of judicial institutions, access typically followed a top-down approach: approval was initially sought from the relevant jurisdictional justice or security departments, followed by authorisation from the prison directors. In some cases, however, access was achieved more informally through participation in open events such as workshops, theatre performances, or sports matches. These events provided opportunities to engage with individuals and assess the feasibility of conducting interviews. Ultimately, in these informal contexts, the 'porous' nature of Latin American prisons, with less stringent controls and more open interactions between inmates and outsiders, allowed for a more adaptable approach to access.

The process of negotiating access to prisons was often highly complex and involved expectations of reciprocity. Institutions more accustomed to academic research generally displayed a better understanding of the logistics and timelines of fieldwork, resulting in more formalised bureaucratic procedures. Conversely, many facilities adopted informal practices, such as issuing visitor or teacher passes to facilitate interviews. Initially, this sometimes included inquiries about potential economic benefits for the prison or offers of services such as lectures or workshops. However, when prison authorities became aware of my specific focus on femicide, their interest in discussing results or organising events often waned.

I interpret this reaction as indicative of the perceived importance—or lack thereof—assigned to femicide, mirroring broader institutional attitudes towards violence against women. Within the moral economy of these prisons, violence against women attracted considerable attention compared to property crimes and drug dealing, for instance. Femicide, like rape, was heavily stigmatised, often implying informal social marginalisation, cyclical punishments, and broader othering practices that separated 'normal' offenders from the 'monstrous'. Nonetheless, for both people in prison and staff alike, there was nothing enigmatic about

[1] For more information about this project, visit www.crimeinlatinamerica.com.

these crimes—not something to be understood, just something to be attacked.

Each prison operated under its own distinct protocols, resulting in varied processes for conducting interviews. In some instances, access was restricted to specific areas, buildings, or rooms. In other cases, I was escorted by security staff as I navigated through the prison corridors. Additionally, there were instances where I received a pass that allowed me, albeit with certain limitations, to move fairly freely within the prison's common areas, such as the corridors, gardens, and educational facilities.

Contact with each participant was primarily facilitated through intermediaries. Initially, prison staff—typically those responsible for maintaining custody records—connected me with men charged with femicide or feminicide (depending on the country). This approach proved most effective, as knowledge of individuals' crimes is often limited within facilities, a practice commonly referred to as not sharing the "first page" (*carátula*) of their files for security reasons. However, in most cases, contacts were established through other individuals encountered during fieldwork, which introduced a bias shaped by the pre-existing relationships and friendships among participants.

To choose the men I interviewed, I followed a convenience sampling approach. While not strictly rigid, I considered factors such as age and educational trajectory to ensure variability within each country. Although this was not quota sampling per se, it allowed me to form a final sample with age and education distributions comparable to those of femicide perpetrators elsewhere.

Interviews were typically conducted in quiet and comfortable settings, such as visitor sections, gardens, classrooms, prison offices, and technical rooms. This choice, both in my own fieldwork and in interviews conducted by others, was intended to create an environment conducive to lengthy and meaningful discussions. While the concept of rapport could be debated due to the inherent power asymmetry between the researcher and people in prison, I found it essential to provide a space that ensured safety from potential threats posed by other prisoners, given the nature of their crimes. Crucially, this approach aimed to minimise the participants' exposure to the watchful gaze of both people in prison and staff (Crewe, 2009). Although this form of surveillance does not require the physical presence of a witness, as it is often internalised, my primary aim was to control the presence of others to ensure a more secure and private interview environment.

The Men

For this book, I analysed 55 life story interviews with men serving prison sentences for femicide/feminicide, conducted over an eight-year period. Of these, I personally conducted 29, while the remaining interviews were carried out by research assistants or colleagues, all working within the same framework. The participants included 20 from Argentina, 15 from Bolivia, 5 from Chile, 2 from Honduras, 4 from Mexico, 7 from Paraguay, and 2 from Venezuela. The uneven distribution of participants primarily reflects the practicalities of fieldwork, such as conducting these interviews alongside other criminological research projects and varying levels of access in different countries. The higher proportion of men from Argentina is largely due to the fact that I carried out a greater number of interviews in my home country.

All the individuals examined in this book are cisgender men who committed intimate femicide or feminicide (depending on local legal definitions) against cisgender women in Latin America. This means they had been specifically charged with that crime, which served as the main inclusion criterion. All were aged 18 or older at the time of the offence. These men were incarcerated for this crime at the time of their initial interview, although some were released over the course of the fieldwork and the process of writing this book. This selection criterion excludes a broader range of cases, omitting men whose victims were trans women, those who killed women who were not intimate partners, and those who committed suicide.

Crucially, all participants incorporated in the analysis of this book admitted to the crime. This is a significant methodological consideration. Academic research, as well as journalistic inquiries, often relies on a state's conviction as the final arbiter of guilt—an approach I find problematic, or at least insufficient, as it typically rests on the unexamined assumption of the state's correctness (Presser, 2013, p. 13). More than anything else, it obscures the methodological transparency we strive to achieve (Di Marco & Rowlands, 2025). To circumvent this issue, I only included men who explicitly acknowledged killing their intimate partners.

In terms of age at the time of the offense, the youngest participant was 21 years old, while the oldest was 68. 15% of perpetrators were aged 21–24, 30% were aged 25–34, 25% were aged 35–44, 20% were aged 45–54, and 10% were aged 55 or older. This relatively homogeneous distribution could be attributed to the sampling criteria. However, the higher proportion of participants in the 25–45 age group may reflect the actual elevated rates of perpetration observed in this age bracket in Latin America (UNODC & UN Women, 2024).

Similarly, the men varied considerably in terms of their formal education prior to imprisonment: 25% had completed no more than primary education, 35% had finished secondary school, 20% had attained some form of tertiary or vocational education (such as technical training in plumbing), and 10% had obtained a university education. Notably, 10% had not completed primary school. Due to the limited number of cases per country, making cross-country comparisons is challenging. However, when grouping educational levels into two broad categories—those with less than secondary education and those with secondary education or above—in general, the sample reveals similar structure across all countries. This distribution broadly aligns with educational attainment rates across Latin America (Arias Ortiz et al., 2024).

The Interviews

> Interviews are sites in which these men can assert their dominance, and in turn, maintain and reproduce gendered patterns of power and authority. (Dheensa et al., 2022, p. 359)

The life stories shared in this book stem from lengthy and often intense conversations with these men, conducted across multiple meetings, typically in sessions lasting 75 minutes, having usually two or three in total. Between these sessions, and while they were still in prison, we engaged in small talk, exchanged updates on our daily lives, shared WhatsApp messages and memes, and remained in contact well beyond the 'fieldwork' phase. These interviews took place over weeks and, in some cases, extended into months of semi-regular dialogue.

The interviews included in this book—whether conducted by other researchers or myself—followed a similar open-ended approach. They were guided by a broad and detailed interview script, serving more as a signpost for thematic domains and a reminder of key aspects rather than a rigid structure. There were no procedural constraints on how the stories were elaborated. This guide and approach were developed in collaboration with Sveinung Sandberg and Gustavo Fondevila for the CRIMLA project, and were generously reviewed by Christoffer Carlsson.

The interviews I personally conducted predominantly employed a narrative technique, encouraging participants to recount their life stories in their own words without imposing a predefined set of questions. This approach was primarily inspired by Gabriele Rosenthal's work (2004). I began by inviting participants to share a spontaneous and detailed narrative of their life events and experiences, with particular emphasis on their romantic relationships. To facilitate their storytelling, I frequently employed clarification ('What does that mean?'), exemplification ('Can you give me an example?'), and paralinguistic cues (such as 'mhm'). My aim was to allow participants to expand their narratives in whichever direction they chose, without imposing any guidance on how or what to share. I adhered to the principle of openness and 'floating attention'—a concept often associated with the psychoanalytic method (Freud, 1977 [1912]). This involved maintaining a receptive stance and allowing participants' thoughts and emotions to unfold, without steering the conversation.

I adopted this open approach, firstly, because it is an optimal way to explore narratives as a practice. This approach assumes that their narratives are intrinsically worthy of analysis. It also challenges the mainstream, naïve notion that this research is about manipulating participants into 'confessing' or devising strategies to deceive them. There was no intention of 'trapping' participants into talking about the crime or disclosing hidden truths about themselves (contrary to what TV shows might suggest about criminological work). Secondly, narration circumvents the problem of simply asking the question 'why' (Bancroft, 2003). Comprehension of shared rationale may be better explored through extended accounts of the self, as Butler argues (2005): stories serve both as vessels for meaning and as objects of significance in their own right.

In all cases, the storytelling unfolded into long, zigzagging conversations over the sessions. The initial sessions were typically free-flowing. The opening questions, designed to trigger narration, combined with the participants' motivation to speak, proved sufficient to elicit detailed accounts. In the final session, departing from the strict narrative approach, I typically explored previously mentioned or missing aspects in greater depth, such as interpersonal conflicts and their sexual and romantic experiences. This session was partly reserved for more "intrinsic questions" (Chaitin, 2004), aimed at clarifying or expanding upon the content that had emerged.

In three instances, I chose to present the entire transcripts to interviewees who had expressed an interest in understanding how their information was being handled and, more specifically, how the data "looked". This interaction also allowed for a deeper understanding—through dialogue—of how they interpreted and, in some cases, contested the transcribed narratives. However, this was not an attempt to validate the veracity or accuracy of the written word.

All sessions were digitally recorded. Initially, I took extensive fieldnotes during the interviews, attempting to capture non-verbal cues, impressions, and analytical memos. This was driven by a prescriptive, generic expectation of what should go into a fieldnote, alongside a desire to document as many details as possible (Elliott & Wolf-Meyer, 2024). However, given the almost artificial and awkward effect that those notes had in face-to-face conversations—especially due to their length—I decided to stop after the first few cases. While note-taking occasionally encouraged participants to speak, as it was perceived as prioritising their words, in many other instances, it became a hindrance.

Agendas

> Certain interviewees did not try to dominate or overpower me but, instead, disarmed me by showing their vulnerabilities. (Robben, 1996, p. 88)

The extensive interviewing process yielded a considerable wealth of written transcripts, which form the core material for analysis here (Fig. 4.1). If one were to visualise the structure of these transcripts, it would resemble a bandoneón or accordion: short questions or interjections from me or the interviewers, followed by lengthy passages of text from the interviewees. This is far from being merely a detail of the fieldwork. Compared to transcripts from interviews with others, such as sex offenders, the men in this study spoke at considerable length, requiring few decisive interventions to encourage their storytelling. Moreover, most of the men contacted were eager to share their stories, with rejection rates, so to speak, being almost negligible across the different prisons and countries. These two points naturally raise intriguing questions: why were they so willing to talk so extensively? Why, despite the paramount stigma in prison surrounding their crime, did men who had killed their partners seem less reluctant to engage? This presents an apparent paradox.

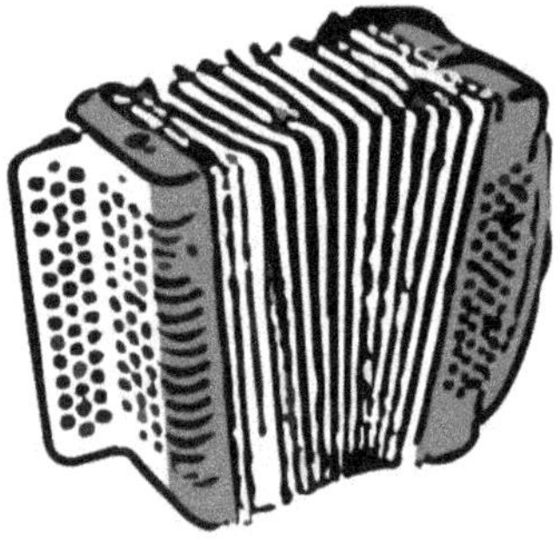

Fig. 4.1 Bandoneón

Most of the men used our encounters to share extensive details about their lives. Some spoke about their children, shared photographs, and delved deeply into harrowing personal experiences. Others remained stoic, avoiding overly emotional portrayals of themselves, yet spoke at length about their relationships. Many also sought my perspective on their situations, seeking validation for the more sensitive statements they made. Most described their relationships with the victim in ways that positioned themselves as distanced from 'actual' culpability.

It should be clear that every person who agrees to talk about their life has their own agenda for doing so. As with any interaction, talking is part of identity construction and a key element of face-to-face communication: we 'become' when talking about ourselves (Tewksbury & Gagné, 2001). Whether they were presenting themselves in a certain light (e.g., as redeemed, solemn, or stoic), seeking recognition, or simply wanting someone to hear them, their reasons for participating inevitably shaped the stories they told.

The eagerness to participate provided the first clue to understanding their narratives. For these men, reclaiming control over the stories told about them seemed crucial. This is even more understandable given the media attention surrounding some cases and the efforts of victims' families and relatives. Distancing themselves from labels like '*femicida*', 'violent', or 'woman killer' was a recurring theme in their conversations and the extensive discussions surrounding these issues. The interviews provided an ideal space for such demonstrations.

This self-presentation is even more understandable when considering the institutional trajectory these men had experienced. Arrests, trials, interactions with the police, radical shifts in their social capital, and, in some cases, media exposure inevitably shaped their accounts. Their presentation of past events was influenced not only by the moment of narration but also by the experiences that occurred between the events and their retelling (Rosenthal, 2018). Given these trajectories, it is clear that, in most cases, their stories have been practiced over months or even years.

However, their interest in speaking about their lives cannot be solely explained by a desire to defend a particular persona. Although the interviews were typically conducted in private settings, they were undoubtedly under the watchful eyes of others in prison, including staff. The "depth" and "weight" of imprisonment (Crewe, 2020), coupled with the consequent observational scrutiny, created an environment of constant spectatorship that affected both the participants and myself. I had anticipated that agreeing to talk to me, and being seen doing so, might disadvantage them in this context, but it was not so straightforward. While some mentioned the risk of retaliation and informal punishment in prison for 'trying to convince' others of their innocence, most appeared to view exposing their truths as advantageous. "I always tell them I have nothing to hide", one interviewee remarked. "This is how I prove it."

Overall, there was little hesitation: firmness in their statements was the norm. For most men, this involved affirming the soundness of their crime or the logic behind it—whether explaining a temporary loss of control or defending their actions. For some, it was a concession of the harm done. In all cases, the explicit reasons given for speaking became clear: telling their stories was strongly motivated by ideas of healing, self-improvement, emotional release, or, most often, offering alternative versions of events.

An analysis of all the agendas at play would require its own book, as this is an ever-present and ongoing aspect of the interview process. I have chosen to address this issue briefly here, as it sets the tone for my analysis of the vignettes. It also aims to place readers in a better position to understand that these life stories, like any other, are not mere narrations of events but engagements with an audience (the interviewers in this case), shaped by agendas, and interpellated by certain themes. Identifying these interpellated themes is key to understanding their narratives.

Vignettes

> It may not be exactly true, but it makes a great story. (Schulman, 1984, p. 41)

Whether in social sciences, literature, investigative journalism, or art, the question of how to represent people has long been of paramount importance (Fig. 4.2). This issue challenges us to consider how to effectively portray individuals and situations, as well as which elements are distinctive. It also raises the question of how much fidelity we owe to the information captured in an MP3 file, a photograph, a notebook, or a court file. Moreover, representation compels many to reflect on the impact such portrayals have on audiences and the extent to which researchers are transparent in the 'translation' process between interlocutors and the written text. As Lawrence-Lightfoot (1997) argues, there seems to be a "science of portraiture".

When it comes to violence, the ethics of evidence becomes even more complex, as we are dealing with a deeply contested issue. Here, ethical dilemmas arise in portraying both the lived experiences of harm (Haines et al., 2019) and its performance (Robben & Hinton, 2023). Ultimately, how to represent becomes very much a moral and political question.

In this book, I use nine vignettes: short life stories selected to illustrate archetypal characteristics of the narratives I have encountered. I use this term to describe the type of textuality I have produced. These vignettes are compositions "in which the features of several research participants are combined into the representative character or exceptional type of person" (Elliott & Wolf-Meyer, 2024, p. 13). These compositions focus on specific elements, such as possessiveness or body terrorism, which I emphasise in the analysis. Thus, it is clear that they should not be

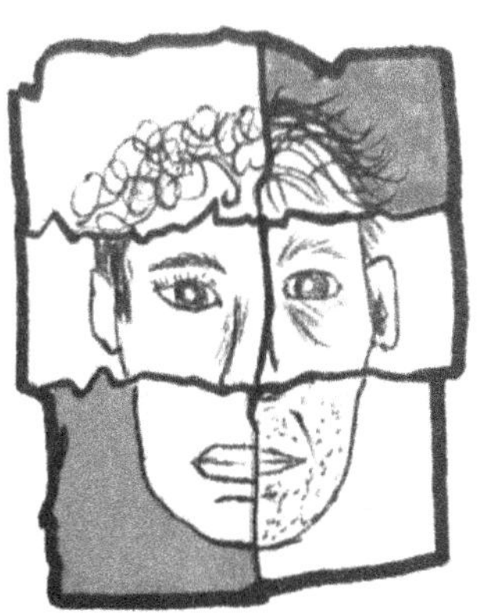

Fig. 4.2 Vignettes

considered life histories (reconstructed a trajectory) or life stories (narratives produced by a teller to convey meaning about past events and to present themselves) per se. They do not aspire to be exhaustive or coherent. A biographical vignette has a shorter format and is shaped by the researcher's analytical process.

In my view, there is no such thing as biographical realism. On the contrary, these cases should remind us of the fictional nature of data. These vignettes, therefore, function as textual products that highlight—rather than obscure—their layers of hermeneutical production: experiential (rooted in the moment of the event), memorial (discursive reconstruction from the present), interactional (shaped contextually and situationally during the interview), and transformative (altered by me through processes of transcription, selection, and rewriting). By foregrounding these interpretive and creative layers, the vignettes serve as a device to challenge biographical illusions (Bourdieu, 2017)—the fallacy of believing that a person's life can be coherently narrated as if it were continuous, linear, and internally consistent. Such illusions impose an artificial sense of order on lives, ignoring the influence of social structures and the unpredictable contingencies that shape individual experiences. In this sense, the vignettes explicitly acknowledge their inherent fictionality.

Vignettes also provide a valuable means of addressing the delicate issues of anonymity and confidentiality. I faced the challenge of offering detailed accounts that captured the nuances and tangible aspects of people's lives while ensuring their identities remained protected. With the increasing media attention on gender-based violence, where cases are often sensationalised in the evening news, the risk of exposure is heightened. These compositions offered an alternative. They also served as a way to reclaim these stories from the media's standardised and reductive narratives, presenting a more nuanced and complex portrayal of the cases.

Composing cases allows for the safeguarding of sensitive data that could reveal participants' vulnerabilities while prioritising the creation of theoretically-driven descriptions. Similarly, Auyero and Swinton (2009), in their cubist ethnography, describe this approach, stating, "the skeptical ethnographer differs from those devoted ethnographers who search for a singular truth. The readiness to integrate contrasting perspectives is crucial to conceptual development" (p. 14). In my work, however, I do not synthesise the views of multiple actors; rather, I construct perspectives derived from a plurality of comparable individuals. Consequently, this approach also highlights commonalities among the men across the region, rather than initiating an inquiry into specific lives—a practice uncritically embraced by mass media.

After completing all the interviews and 'testing' their flexibility in various ways over two years, I decided to adopt this approach for the vignettes. First, I selected the main themes that were both prominent in the conversations with the men and those I wanted to present in the book. The nine vignettes address, each with its own nuances, three overarching topics: rule-breaking (expectations, punishment, and control); social relationships and contexts (peer support, neighbourhood reliability, and institutional navigation); and the contextualisation of stories (institutional discourses, blatant misogyny, and chaotic narratives). Next, I classified the cases that initially provided the empirical grounding for these themes and selected specific life events that could be assembled (for instance, descriptions of childhood) based on similarities between cases and within each theme. I preserved the sequences each individual used in their accounts, adhering to their natural logic in narrating events: for example, accounts of femicide often preceded childhood narratives, and descriptions of life in prison generally came before details of their trials. More often than not, I also used their own terms to discuss events, people, and emotions.

These vignettes merge parts of stories based on empirical similarities across cases (e.g., shared descriptions of first romantic relationships) and analytical relevance (e.g., themes that equally illustrate bodily control and coercion). This approach helped further obscure identities, as a standard biographical technique (Plummer, 1995, p. 7). Ultimately, this strategy was designed to preserve the coherence of each case (i.e., the shared aspects among the men) while also protecting individual identities (Witte, 2016).

In keeping with mainstream traditions in anthropology, I employed the words and expressions used by the interviewees during our discussions. Naturally, the translation into English somewhat diluted this strategy. Nevertheless, I believe that preserving the emic wording adds nuance and plurality to the vignettes. After all, the story of a 60-year-old engineer is, understandably, different from that of a 21-year-old manual worker.

Ethics

Ethical challenges are, ultimately, practical ones. They are neither categorical, Kantian black-and-white situations nor merely bureaucratic concerns about transparency, data storage, and potential risks. Rather, they involve the decisions we make throughout the research process and even after its completion (Guillemin & Gillam, 2004). This may seem counterintuitive, especially in the social sciences, where research is often perceived as innocuous. Yet working with imprisoned individuals who have caused harm laid bare the highly sensitive nature of this endeavour. From grappling with the implications of learning about unreported crimes (e.g., Bourgois, 2003; Noel, 2011) to providing a platform for those who have inflicted harm (Robben & Hinton, 2023), and obtaining informed consent while safeguarding their privacy in publications, ethical considerations become profoundly complex.

Ironically, the first ethical challenge emerged in my interactions with ethics review boards across two countries, which evaluated the project. Primarily, these arose during the first rounds of feedback. I received comments—some of which could be interpreted as objections—regarding the study's purpose: Why is it relevant? How can interviewing perpetrators contribute valuable academic knowledge? Will this not simply justify their actions? This led to a protracted exchange of comments, revisions, and additional feedback.

This exchange can be interpreted as part of a broader reluctance to endorse or validate studies focused on those who harm. I perceived this as a somewhat misguided attempt to question the purpose of biographical research, defaulting towards a stance of complete ostracisation or demonisation of perpetrators, while also attempting to constrain qualitative research within the frameworks of other scientific traditions. However, this may be an unfair reading; these interactions could have been the result of a genuine concern with the utility of the research. Nonetheless, the thorny process of navigating multiple ethics boards underscored that ethical considerations extend beyond institutional guidelines and reflect the highly contested nature of this topic—where punishment often takes precedence over the development of prevention strategies.

Reflecting on the main aims of this research made me consider how the book might be seen as a sordid, voyeuristic portrayal of violence. This concern was also raised by several actors during fieldwork, including the families of the victims. The prevalence of what has been termed a pornography of violence (Bourgois, 2003) and penal spectatorship (Brown, 2013), even within narrative criminology (Bunn, 2023), heightened this concern. I was particularly mindful of this issue. Undoubtedly, it redirected attention to my reasons for writing this book.

There are, I believe, two primary imperatives for pursuing perpetrator-focused research on femicide. First, it is essential to build theories of femicide that account for the actual rationalities of perpetrators, rather than assumptions made about them. This was the initial impetus for this research and it remained relatively unchanged throughout the process. However, conversations along the way reinforced a second motivation: our collective interventions against violence can be informed by these stories—though the ways in which they can be integrated into policy and practice may not be straightforward or easily systematised. Examining the 'black box' of perpetration is, I believe, an unavoidable step in this process. Viewing academic work on perpetrators from this perspective provides valuable insights, countering overly broad critiques of spectatorship when disconnected from practical applications. A more cynical reading might correctly highlight the utility of writing a book as a means of career advancement within the academic marketplace. This is a valid and realistic parallel aspect of the project.

The issue of protecting participants from harm arose as a key concern during the project. Participation had layers of impact on the lives of these men, whose daily routines were highly institutionalised. Many were blacklisted by both the penal system and other prisoners and were regarded as the most morally condemnable. Simply being seen in open spaces or talking with an outsider (often assumed to be justifying themselves to the media) could put them at risk. Stories of torture circulate regularly as moralising tales among inmates. This situates us in a different position from radical perspectives which argue that our moral duty to victims of injustice outweighs our commitment to professional ethical codes (Scheper-Hughes, 1995). While understandable given the uneven power structures and stark epistemic injustices involved, I do not adopt such a stance. My position is not based on regarding this approach as intrinsically problematic but rather on seeing it as unproductive for understanding violence.

For my fieldwork, this meant having a clear alert system: if I perceived or was informed of danger to participants, I would stop interviews. In some cases, it also involved coordinating with authorities for specific protective measures, such as changing facilities. Although more a precaution than an actual trend, this demonstrated how even a 'simple' qualitative project could endanger participants, forcing us to confront the paradox of protecting those who have caused harm, regardless of personal moral views.

The issue of anonymity arose not only with ethics boards but also in the handling of data and writing projects. With recognisable events and details, the challenge of 'blurring' identities while maintaining empirical accuracy became central. To address this, I used pseudonyms for people, streets, cities, towns, and institutions. When professions or personal traits were too revealing, I substituted them with comparable alternatives, such as replacing 'engineer' with 'architect.' I also reconstructed significant events, such as weddings being reframed as birthday parties, and mixed popular first names from different countries to prevent inference of each character's origin. Since these measures alone were insufficient, creating composite vignettes became essential to ensure anonymity while preserving the integrity of the narratives.

Reflecting on how to maintain anonymity in my writing led to a broader question about writing itself. As a non-native English speaker, I am acutely aware of the delicate political nature of choosing which language to use. In Latin America, Spanish serves as the lingua franca in most of the region—a legacy of colonialism. Writing in English, however, aims to expand the topic of femicide—deeply connected with the Latin American context—to other regions, where discussions of domestic homicide have developed less politically charged tones. While translating the words of the interviewed men homogenises their speech and erases traces of local lexicon, it also facilitates anonymity and highlights general patterns across the region. This decision, I hope, is understood by discerning readers as an effort to foster broader understanding.

There is an additional risk that extends beyond the book itself: the individualisation of the femicide perpetration. This work is grounded in the idea that the narratives I discuss are not individual in origin, nor are they merely the result of psychological issues (though such factors may exist). Interpreting the 'monstrosity' of men reverts us to a narrow view of violence more generally. Femicide is not an issue confined to these men and women; it is a societal issue that affects us all.

Fieldwork also brought significant internal conflicts on a personal level. Conducting the interviews was not a Herculean task; most conversations unfolded without drama or unexpected revelations and were neither terrifying nor particularly moving. Yet, the writing phase became increasingly uncomfortable and emotionally taxing, as it underscored an extreme form of victim silencing and profound hermeneutic injustice: while the men's voices were foregrounded, the voices of the women remained absent and unheard.

Beyond Fieldwork

I have reserved this section for last, in which I address 'going public' as discussed by Sanjek (2004) in relation to publications and communications, as it serves as a fitting preface to the vignettes and the contexts in which they were produced.

Logically, the individuals most immediately affected by the publication of research are the participants themselves. I initially anticipated a stronger, perhaps harsher, reaction from participants to whom I had shared feedback, articles, or other dissemination outputs. However, they often neither empathised with nor identified with the texts. Discussions around narratives, discourses, emotions, and, in some cases, personal histories, appeared to them as topics relevant only to the 'actual' group of femicide perpetrators—the 'real' perpetrators, the 'crazy' ones, the 'evil' ones—terms they themselves used to refer to such individuals, not to themselves. This response reveals much about the difficulty of acknowledging perpetrated violence.

Other men contacted me after reading some text, usually from media coverage. This not only served as a reminder that participants do, in fact, read our work, but also that their interpretations are often shaped by their own agendas and how the published text might affect their perceived identities. I would say that, in most cases, they were primarily concerned that their specific stories were not heard. Their accounts of innocence or the 'real' version of events did not come across as they had expected.

In other cases, conversations sparked by papers or news articles led to direct confrontations with the text. These ranged from perceiving the publication as inaccurate in relation to their experiences ("This has nothing to do with what I told you. It's all wrong", one interviewee said) to feeling specifically offended by certain terms, notably 'violence'. Given that key issues in these narratives often revolve around aggression, responsibility, and motivation, these tensions are understandable. As Scheper-Hughes (1992) notes, the disclosure of truths can strain the balance between the perspectives held by researchers and those held by research participants. In this case, the balance seemed to be most affected when violence was referenced, when bidirectional violence was not represented, or when they did not see their actions portrayed as 'understandable'.

Abu-Lughod (2008) captures this tension well by stating: "One of the challenges of writing about people who may read what you write is the ethical and intellectual responsibility to represent them in ways that they might recognise and find truthful." The challenge is even greater in this case, where the subject of representation (murder) and, more specifically, its underlying causes, remain highly contested.

Paradoxically, bringing this to light in a book entails a difficult conversation about the exposure of our texts and their impact on participants. More importantly, it highlights the situation of these men after imprisonment and the lack of institutional avenues for their 'treatment.' I hypothesise that, in a different institutional context during their time in prison, their reactions might have been different. They could have been more likely to acknowledge their violence, less inclined to 'other' the aggression, and more willing to engage with researchers from a different perspective. Given that most participants agreed to take part in the study in order to tell their side of the story and reclaim a positive persona, a different institutional scenario that placed more emphasis on their treatment might actually have disincentivised them from opening up to outsiders.

Some feminist organisations, as well as NGOs supporting victims' families and survivors, understandably critiqued my work—and the broader line of inquiry on perpetration—viewing it as morally contentious. Working with perpetrators meant crossing a moral boundary: some accepted it without endorsement, while others dismissed it outright as a "waste of time, effort, and funds". For some, focusing on men felt like a betrayal, as allocating resources to them could detract from other areas of the field. This stance inevitably led to closed doors and rivalries, which, in my view, fragmented rather than strengthened our collective cause. Additionally, my identity as a white Latino cis man leading the project was criticised: "It is shameful to see a man talking about femicide", one person commented during a YouTube live-streamed presentation in Mexico. Accusations of insensitivity were an extension of this moral judgement.

I consider work with perpetrators essential for understanding and preventing harm. As in any fieldwork, researchers must establish and maintain rapport, which includes creating comfort, demonstrating empathy without judgement, and signalling certain forms of respect with participants. Yet, as Dheensa et al. (2022) argue, balancing these principles becomes a challenge when competing aims and values are involved in working with these men.

Ultimately, this may be a question of proximity to the task itself. Nils Christie (1981) captured this concept so aptly that it seems fitting to reference his words directly:

> The seriousness of the core phenomena within penal law is easily forgotten. If an employee in a funeral bureau allowed themselves to become involved with all the sorrow they encountered, if they took it on and in themselves, they might soon have to change their occupation. The same is likely true for those of us who work in, or are closely connected

with, the penal law system. The questions confronting us are difficult to live with. We survive by turning the work into routine, by engaging with only small bits of the totality at a time, and by distancing ourselves from the client, particularly from the client's experience of their own situation. (p. 13)

Part II

Listening to Their Stories

5 Safeguarding Gender Norms

Safeguarding gender norms was a recurring theme in the conversations with the interviewed men. This involved discussions about their rigid dos and don'ts: how women should dress, behave, where they should be, and how they should love. They also spoke about expectations for their own behaviour and that of other men. Men and women were invariantly treated as 'objects' in their discourse. As stories go, this was not surprising. I took this morality-packed discourse as an initial gateway to navigate their narratives and identify some recurring themes.

These moral imperatives were, however, not always neatly presented in our conversations; they were often camouflaged in anecdotes, justifications, and reflections. Additionally, the men told their stories in various ways: sometimes clearly trying to present a respectable narrative, and other times carelessly venting their emotions. The tricky part was to remember that, regardless of the content or delivery, the men were presenting their self in what Goffman (1956) classically called the presentation of a virtual persona: much like actors on a stage, performing roles in social interactions, adjusting their behaviour to manage impressions and achieve desired outcomes.

M. H. Di Marco, *Narratives of Femicide Perpetrators in Latin America*,
https://doi.org/10.1007/978-3-031-97367-3_5

In these stories, defying certain norms often led to conflict-ridden—and usually emotionally catastrophic—scenarios. Sometimes rule-breaking was linked to the functioning of a household, other times to the dissolution of a relationship. Occasionally, it was about more ephemeral topics, such as expectations for a birthday party. My deliberate approach was to explore the implications of these rule-breaking stories, no matter how minuscule or seemingly irrelevant they might seem. In so doing, I realised that violating gender norms was always at the epicentre of femicide. Regardless of the women's actions, the men's suspicions, feelings of threat, and fear (a psychologist might label this paranoia) were unavoidable components in understanding their behaviour.

In this chapter, I present three vignettes that illustrate how men's perceptions of gender norms are central to understanding their expressions of wrath. Jorge, Celso, and Héctor share deeply ingrained notions of moral boundaries—the implicit rules and expectations that define acceptable behaviour and relationships within their social and cultural frameworks. In the interviews, they reconstruct how the violation of certain norms—such as those surrounding domestic duties, fidelity, and loyalty—was perceived as a direct and defiant threat to their identities as men. These moments of transgression exposed the moral rules underpinning their worldview and revealed the fragile dynamics at play when such boundaries are challenged.

Jorge: The Birthday Cake

Jorge met Sabrina in a local night club: they stared at each other all night long and, just before the night ended, he finally plucked up the courage to talk to her (Fig. 5.1). They started dating right away and spent the first seven months in what he described as "blissful happiness". At the time, he was 22 and she was 18:

> It's hard to explain, but I felt we were made for each other. Not the silly joke where we ended each other's sentences. But everything fitted. We liked each other, we made each other laugh. It was like we had a similar pace in life, so things worked smoothly. I had just ended a relationship

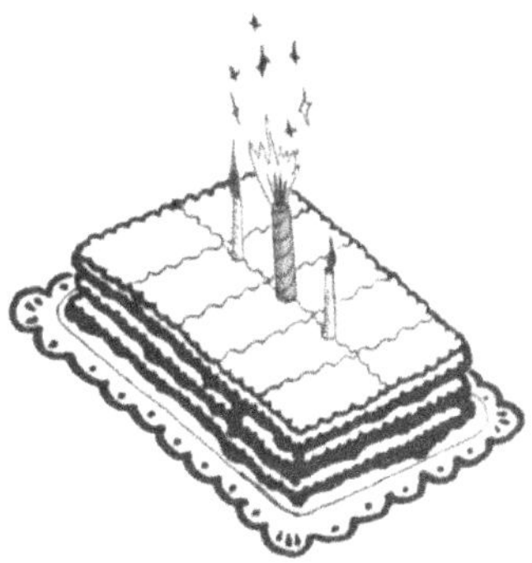

Fig. 5.1 Chocotorta

> before, so she made me move forward. And I was her first boyfriend. [Silence]. I knew right away we were made for each other: there had been no one else in my life who made me feel so calm and reassured.

Both Jorge and Sabrina had similar social backgrounds. They were born and raised in the outskirts of the capital and spent most of their lives in the same town. Their daily routines revolved around places and people they knew since infancy. Their families were working class and had been deeply affected by the national economy's ups and downs. In his words, both experienced being "locked up in the same labyrinth". This shared experience brought them closer, as they both understood the struggles of life on the periphery.

They moved in together a year after they met. He wanted to settle down and she was struggling to have a peaceful life while living with her mother and abusive stepfather. Their relationship had always been stormy, and during the last months Sabrina lived in the house, physical aggression between her and her stepfather became frequent:

> I guess moving in was a normal step for any couple. We needed our own space, and to build our project following our own rules, you know? So I found this small flat, right above a vehicle repair shop. One bedroom, living room. Good enough for two. It was more or less close to my neighbourhood. A bus on the main avenue would take us to my parents' house. So then we moved in.

Jorge describes the following years as "normal"—a word used frequently in our conversations. After moving in, he started working in the vehicle repair shop below their flat and began attending classes to become a certified mechanic. He also wanted to start a family with her and settle down. During this time, she was working as a cashier in the local butcher's shop. While they had always struggled to make ends meet, he was reluctant to state that she needed to work as well:

> I think we could have managed with my salary. It was not much, but we could have. But she wanted to have her own money. Of course, I understand that. This changed later, when the abortion happened.

A year after they had moved in together, she got pregnant. Having children was something they had discussed before, but she remained unsure and apprehensive. The idea reminded her of her own torturous childhood. Jorge, on the other hand, saw parenthood as a normal step in their relationship. Sabrina found out about her pregnancy and decided to end it without telling him. This moment was a landmark in his story: it signalled a radical change in his attitude towards her:

> I came home one day. It was Friday. And she was waiting for me in the kitchen, sitting down. I noticed she had been weird that last week, but she wouldn't tell me what was going on. But I trusted her until that point. Then she asked me to sit down and told me she had an abortion. An abortion of a child I never even knew I was having. She decided, on her own, she didn't want to have our child.

There was a crescendo to Jorge's tone and the rhythm of his words grew faster. He was successfully transmitting despair and anger in the interview. The "unilateral abortion", as he called it, was unshakeable, and unforgivable:

> I felt betrayed, I felt stabbed in the back and defiled. My blood pressure dropped when she uttered abortion. I almost fainted. I couldn't believe what was happening. Was she really telling me she had killed our unborn child? Then, I exploded. I was so, so furious.

For the first time in his account, Jorge mentioned physical violence. Shielded by the idea that he was completely "out of himself", he described beating her and smashing the kitchen table. Not only had she killed an innocent child, but she had also completely disregarded *his* desires. As he recounted this moment, it became evident that, in his mind, the violence was a justifiable response.

The relationship was stained by this event and, in the following year, he became increasingly violent. In his words, he became more "temperamental". Bouts of arguments, feeling unhappy and slapping her were followed by moments of calmness and tenderness. Jorge was aware of this new cycle: he suffered the moments of conflict and felt unable to change his own attitudes:

> I was conscious of all of this. Well, not in [he stressed] each fight, but every weekend after a big conflict, I would think: what the fuck happened? Perhaps it was because I was not working those days and I had time to reflect. But that is how things worked, because when we fought, I was unaware of it. And then the guilt kicked in.

Jorge started our third interview by talking about the last year of the relationship. By that time, he was 34 and she was 30. Compared to the "normal" years at the start of their relationship, this last year was marked by deep emotional turmoil. Jorge felt a constant inner conflict: he was unable to control himself, fights were cyclical and he saw them happen in slow motion:

> I never thought of going to therapy, because it was never an actual option. I've heard about psychologists, but it was something for other people. Never actually occurred to me that I needed one. But I was feeling wrong, like there was something wrong. [...]. It's like she had unleashed a part of me that I didn't like, and that took control of my being.

All these changes in his life were accompanied by a period of severe conflicts at work. The opening of new scrapyards near the repair shop had transformed the market and attracted competitors to the area. This dire situation had altered his mood and overall outlook on life.

By the end of that year, he will have murdered Sabrina:

> At some point, we sat down and talked. We were both hurting each other. We knew it, but it seemed we were drawn to these intense fights, and didn′t have the resources, let's say, to do anything about them. I didn't want to separate, she didn't either. I can't remember how it started, but at some point she decided to study to become a kindergarten teacher.

By the way he spoke, Jorge hinted that this was 'the last stage' of their relationship. She enrolled in a local institution to become a teacher, which changed the usual dynamics they had. She was attending classes, meeting new people and making friends. She was still working part-time at the butcher's shop, and attending classes in the afternoon. Her studies introduced a new element to the story, namely, her friends. Until this point in our interviews, Sabrina was implicitly described as isolated. She wanted to steer clear of her family, but he had not mentioned friends of any kind.

Now, her classmates started to enter the picture. They were typically referred to as a source of change and, in some cases, conflict. María, for instance, was Sabrina's closest friend in class. They had become confidants, which did not sit well with Jorge:

> She had different interests. She was younger [19], so she was only interested in partying and meeting guys. Sabrina was in another moment in life. So, when she tried to lure her into her habits, you know, I stood up. It was not even study-related [smirks]. She was just a messy chaos.

While Jorge's disapproval of María was made clear, it did not provoke a major conflict. However, a male classmate, Javier, was another story. Sabrina and Javier became friends in an introductory course, and they attended the same evening class:

> J: This is not about me being jealous, believe it or not [smiles]. This is about her seeking attention: she discovered this new side of her, a tease, probably from this girl María: to tease me, to push me a bit. And of course, of course [raises voice], she had to take an evening class with the only guy in the entire course. I think it was an attempt to provoke me.
> M: Why would she provoke you?
> J: Who knows? Women are complicated sometimes.

Jorge did not want to elaborate on this point. It seems that just accusing her of intentionally making him feel "uneasy" was reason enough to explain both of their attitudes.

By November, conflicts were the order of the day. Sabrina started skipping classes because, as Jorge explained, she was troubled by their relationship. He also mentioned the teachers' high standards. Yet I could not help but think that it was to hide the bodily lacerations of his battering.

December arrived, and so did Jorge's birthday. Ever since he was a child, the expectation to have a birthday party was huge. He would book a venue far in advance, make a guest list, buy as much beer and fernet as he could. For him, it was a moment of joy and the culmination of having 'survived another year':

> Only God knows why I get… got so excited for my birthdays. But I never wanted something very special. You know, normal things in life. A nice party, a good meal, a birthday cake. And she knew it. We spent many birthdays together, and she knew it. I remember asking her for a cake I loved when we were first dating, because I knew she was a great baker.

By the end of December, Sabrina was facing the final exams for her course. She also had to prepare a colloquium, which was a topic of frequent conflict. She was devoting a lot of energy and attention to her studies, at the expense of the relationship. Her studies, the new friendships and the overall change in their "normal" lives were, at this point of the story, paramount obstacles:

> That day, I went to work, before she woke up. I went, had a normal day. And, again, I had never asked for much. But this was important. I got home and she was still not there. There was nothing in the fridge, so I assumed she had hidden the cake in the neighbour's house, so that it would be a surprise. The year before she made this huge [extends his arms] chocolate cake. But she arrived at eight with a bag. She had bought a cake in the shitty pastry shop we had in the neighbourhood. A fucking store-bought cake. That is no way to treat me. I am not an animal [raises voice]. I am not an animal!

He repeated that last statement during our last interview. “This is not a proper way to treat your partner”, “I felt miserable”, “She knew, how couldn’t she?”. It seems clear that the meaning of the birthday cake surpassed its role in the birthday ritual: it spoke to a strikingly normative aspect of their relationship. By buying a cake, instead of baking it, she unknowingly changed a fundamental element of their bond. As with the abortion, Jorge interpreted that this ‘unilateral’ decision was a violation of her role and a direct attack on his person.

As he continued describing the scene, he highlighted his bodily experience in that moment:

> I don’t know. I explained this a million times, but I just snapped. No self-control, no reason. I just snapped, with pure aggression. I do not know if she did this willingly or not. But my body, let’s say, reacted like that. I just shattered into pieces. I was not myself.

Jorge strangled her in the kitchen, next to the birthday cake laying on the countertop. The police arrived, after the owner of the repair shop heard the screams. It was the first time he had intervened.

Over the course of our encounters, the connection between that final fight and the earlier conflicts was never a settled topic. At times, he seemed to intertwine the relationship with the event, as though one flowed inevitably into the other. At other times, he split them apart, presenting two distinct narratives that stood in uneasy isolation. Yet, whenever he revisited that final moment, his account circled back to the same familiar references: a lack of bodily control, fragmented memories, and a sudden, unthinking reaction. These were the only explanations he could muster, fragile threads in a story that remained incomplete.

* * *

Killing a partner for a birthday cake seems almost preposterous. As Kate Manne (2020, p. 18) argues, it can be tempting “to dismiss this [violence] rant and its ilk as the ravings of lunatics”. Indeed, cartoon villain monologues often appear absurd, almost comical. This absurdity, however, is not a sufficient reason to disregard them. The ludicrous emphasis on the cake highlights a crucial element in Jorge’s coda. In the story he recounted, unmet expectations led to escalations in violence. In other words, the discrepancy between his expectations and Sabrina's actions, as well as his sense of entitlement, and his perceived control culminated in femicide.

Unfortunately, many other men share equally absurd stories. Feeling they have nothing left to lose, they may plan to go out in a maximally violent outburst. The common thread is a shift in their expectations. When these expectations go unmet, they often respond by breaking rules. Confronted with situations they find unacceptable, their frustration points to the violation of a tacit norm. For Jorge, this might include everything from his partner studying and having male friends, to working independently and climbing the social ladder. For other men, this clash of expectations might be linked to feelings abandoned or excluded from certain decisions. In all cases, however, unmet expectations were an integral part of their femicidal acts.

Celso: Upholding the Truth

- M: Would you like me to use any particular pseudonym?
- C: No. I have never been afraid of anything.
- M: How so?
- C: No, I have never been afraid of anything in my life.
- M: Never?
- C: No… I have always walked in life upholding the truth.
- M: Upholding the truth, OK. Would you like to tell me a bit about yourself?
- C: Well, my name is Celso. Thirteen years ago, I killed my wife.

Celso, as many other interviewees, presented himself in a stoic, yet sorrowful manner: there was nothing to hide, his crime deserved no shame, and the interview could (and should) have his real name (Fig. 5.2). Readers all over the world should be aware of the actual circumstances of the killing, the true nature of the events.

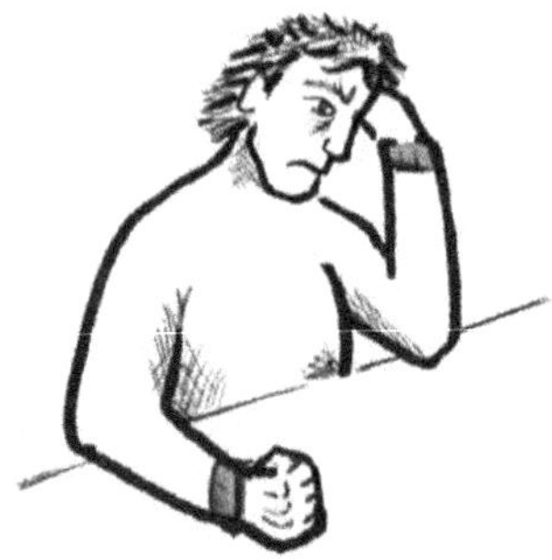

Fig. 5.2 Haunted and worried

He started his story by talking about his relationship with his wife. In a few concise words, he synthesised the ideas that he would later develop in our conversations:

> We had a nice marriage, but... she started misbehaving, very badly. The resentment started piling up... I still love this woman. But we almost had twenty-nine years of marriage... She had two children from different men, I didn't mind that.

Celso grew up with both of his parents and his eight siblings. Raised in a working-class family in a rural area, his parents were not very present during his childhood. They spent most of their time working, and his siblings (most of them his senior) pursued their own hobbies, developed their own skills to take care of themselves and related separately with their own peers.

From a young age, Celso spent a lot of time by himself. As he explained, he liked roaming around the small town. Having an "idle life" was his way of passing time:

> I used to make my parents suffer. I liked the lazy lifestyle. They would send me to buy bread in the morning, and I wouldn't be back before the night. I liked being idle like that. [...]. It was just who I was. I was not even looking for something, doing something bad, or trying to meet people. I just like that.

Celso describes his father as a hardworking man who provided for the entire family. In his view, his father was the pillar of the family: a man who did not argue, who did not fight, and who was focused on working and supporting his family financially. His mother, however, was portrayed in a different light. Although Celso did not express much emotion when talking about her (there was no anger, humour, irony, or resentment in his tone), he emphasised her 'temper':

> She would wait for me to wake up, because I used to get home so late. And she would beat me up. It was my doing though. I was always loitering. [...]. I liked laziness, idleness. So she would beat me up. My father would wait with her. She would punish me.

The few descriptions that Celso provided of his childhood were related to forms of humiliation: from a very young age, he was physically abused, mocked, and criticised. Still, he never referred to these events as painful or scarring in any way. Instead, he would depict them as unrelated events, which had no consequence on himself, his family or, later, the crime he committed.

Although he did not mention his siblings much during his story (they had no names, ages or specific descriptions), an elder brother was mentioned during a particular anecdote. Referring to Celso, this brother asked their father: "Would you have ever guessed this crazy fuck up would get married?!" His father nodded.

Celso did not mention many romantic or sexual partners during his teenage years. He started dating later in life. "I was happy dating women. Nothing serious, just dating, just dating. I was happy like that. I was not in any relationship, so I could do whatever I wanted. But I never dated many women." When I asked him about previous girlfriends, he briefly mentioned one: Jazmin. Their relationship was marked by her job and how, in his mind, it was an obstacle to pursuing a deeper bond:

> But I dated her briefly, because I used to take her to work, and she would never reply when she was there. That relationship ended, to this day, it ended without any explanation. I used to tell her to meet in the main square, but the relationship did not last.

A few years later, Celso met Javiera. She had just given birth to her second child. In our interviews, the introduction of Javiera in his story was connected to her having children with other men:

> I love her and I thought about her children. I thought about them, because they are not guilty of having been born. I have known them since they were small kids. I took the responsibility, but… I made the decision of staying with her, because I love her and I wanted to give her children a future. I took them as my own. One was six, the other one was barely a few months old, and I took them. I don't regret it, because what I was doing was good. I met her with children and I once told her that with those two it was enough, because I didn't have a professional career, I had always worked in construction.

The fact that she had two children from two previous partners was something that Celso highlighted repeatedly in our conversations: he stressed, over and over again, that this was not a problem for him. In an almost charitable fashion, he took them in.

If her children were not a problem, Javiera's attitude certainly was. He repeatedly called her a flirt. Yet unlike accepting her children—something that he had "chosen" to do—, her apparent provocative attitude was her decision. "I was not a jealous man, she made me jealous. I was not jealous, why would I be?"

Celso never provided many details about how they met, if they had mutual friends or if she was still in a relationship at the time. Nonetheless, he mentioned they shared a common faith: they were both devoted Jehova Witnesses.

They dated for three months before getting married in the late 1970s. A few years later, their only child was born. Celso did not describe the years after their marriage or the upbringing of their child. It seems that this stage was unimportant compared to what happened later in their relationship.

In 1988, she told him that she had had an affair with a physician. She met her lover after suffering a severe injury. He was married as well. Celso's life changed drastically: in his words, life turned into a "torment." Most of our conversations revolved around this event. Her 'betrayal'—at least in his story—became a pivotal event that marked him. Having a child and the death of three of his siblings paled in comparison.

In his mind, being single and being in a relationship are two morally distinct situations. He lectured me several times in our meetings. "If you are single, you can date as much as you want. You can have all the fun you want. But if you are committed, no. I will never accept that". This difference was equally universal for men and women: everyone should behave according to this principle, no matter what.

In his story, her confession triggered the only moment in their lives in which physical violence was present, aside from the femicide itself. "I was never again violent after that. Because she behaved badly. She had behaved badly."

His story did not emphasise his violent reaction that day. While he mentioned becoming rageful, it seems his aggression was not as important as the insults he levelled at her. Celso repeated this word—"insults"—over and over again: they were present day and night; he kept blaming her, discrediting her.

Celso had always been jealous and suspicious of her. "Jealousy doesn't appear out of the blue; it has a reason," he said. The confession of infidelity confirmed his suspicions. After this event, he lived in constant tension, torn between feeling pain and deciding whether to stay with her. "I loved her, so I stayed with her. I took care of her. But she betrayed me; she was evil and bad for me. Insults, insults, insults all the time." He denied any form of physical aggression. In his mind, there were only insults, which, to him, were a greater burden than they were to her:

> I remembered… and that was the worst, but I could not leave her, because… because I still love her, I could not leave her, leave our children, because who will take care of them? Me? I was between a rock and a hard place. I had to make a decision… and I stayed with her. I still love her.

I was intrigued by his use of the present tense: he still loves her. While this was not the first time that one of the men I interviewed expressed himself in the present tense, it caught my attention that he recurrently framed his emotions in that way. I asked him about what love meant for him. He was puzzled. "A little bug bites you… you fall in love, you want to get married, start a family, in spite of the fact that… that family… I destroyed it."

As with most of his life story, Celso was not clear with his sequence of events and skipped many years. There was no reference to his children growing up, his job, any friends. Later he resumed the interview with another biographical landmark: a suspected infidelity. Javiera was getting their kitchen painted by a neighbour and Celso was suspicious of the painter:

> She was befriending this painter. I believe in friendship, but when male friends seek the opportunity to be alone with a female friend, it is hard. I do not know in other cases, but I was not smart enough to understand what was going on. I was not smart enough! [...]. It all brought back memories of 1988. She was doing it again, she was doing it again. And I couldn't accept it.

In his mind, their relationship was tainted by the previous conflict: it had changed how they related and, most importantly, how he saw her. "She had a record of… How would you call this? I call it being a flirt. She was very smart, she knew how to make me jealous." Celso repeated the same formula over and over again: "she knew how to make me jealous."

A Friday afternoon, Celso came back home and could not find Javiera. She was visiting the neighbour. When she came back, he "reacted": "I could not help it any longer. I reacted to her teasing, her constant teasing and flirtation. She was not doing me good." He could not contain the anger any longer: he was sure she was cheating on him again.

His eldest stepson, who was 11 years old at that time, found them and called the police.

Celso did not talk about the killing itself. He digressed, changed the topic, and described other events from that day (the weather, his feelings, the architecture of the house). He also seemed unable to talk about how sure he was about the alleged affair. Yet, he was eager to talk about what he did after the femicide: he stabbed himself seven times. Celso showed me his wounds during our last conversation. The showing of scar tissue was a ritual I was privy to on numerous occasions: other men had also shown me the physical lacerations of their 'love' as a way to communicate that they had also experienced sorrow and sadness.

Celso had been in prison for 12 years when we met. Unlike other men, he did not deny the crime, the aggression in the relationship and the constant verbal abuse he inflicted on his wife. On the contrary, he unproblematically talked about his behaviour. But, in doing so, he sought to justify his actions. "I am a delinquent. I don't forgive myself and I will never do it. But she was doing something wrong."

During our last interview, we discussed other men who had committed the same crime and the possibility of change and 'rehabilitation'. It was common for most men to distinguish themselves from other men charged with femicide: they presented their situation as unique, incomparable, and irreducible to a label. This, so far, has been a fairly consistent aspect across all the countries. Celso also attempted to distance himself, but in a less explicit and impactful way:

> It is not very nice what I will say, but… they might do it again, they do it again. I won't, what more could I do? I am a criminal, due to the damage that I inflicted upon my children, to our family, and my grandchildren, but… when she cheated on me, it really marked my life. It was different from that moment onwards.

* * *

My conversations with Celso stand out because of his distinctive way of telling his story. His reminiscing and narrating were marked by a pattern of repetition. Unlike other men, he frequently returned to the same anecdotes, ruminating over them. His storytelling was almost cyclical. The day his wife told him about the affair was a touchstone in his narrative, recurrently described throughout our conversations. It seemed that every moment of his life was connected to this pivotal event; every path led back to that turning point.

Celso was not an eloquent storyteller. He often struggled to find words to describe situations, people, and feelings. Frequently, he would stop mid-sentence, hesitate, and repeat what he had already said. This had a noticeable impact on the flow of his storytelling. This second aspect extends beyond Celso's case and raises a key question about the nature of interviews in general.

Despite the specific character of Celso's storytelling, his narrative shares the core elements I commonly found in femicide stories. Control and possession emerge as constant backdrops against which the relationship is framed. Without understanding the concepts of ownership and entitlement (often referred to as proprietariness), it is challenging to grasp the main plot of this story. Additionally, Celso's lengthy preaching of sexist morals, where he spent considerable time expounding on the essence of faithfulness, underscores his strong sense of righteousness. Ultimately, femicide may be seen as a product of aggrieved entitlement (Kimmel, 2019): the perception of not receiving a certain privilege is interpreted as unfair treatment. Celso feels wronged and sees himself as the victim of a great injustice.

It is worth remembering that the bending of these moral rules represents a 'turning point' in their stories. Traditionally, these are defined as significant events in a person's life that lead to a major change in their sense of self or trajectory (Denzin, 1989). Without understanding this, these pivotal moments are difficult to interpret. Celso repeatedly returns to an alleged infidelity and his 'heroic' acceptance of his pregnant partner, viewing these as indelible moments that stained their relationship. Ultimately, his story follows a tragic arc, where his perceived damage fuels his emotions, justifies his actions, and casts him as the victim.

Héctor: Controlling Her Body

> No one will understand that I still love her—Héctor.

I met Héctor in the plant room of a prison. His cellmates had spoken about him: he was the "wife-killer" of the unit (Fig. 5.3). They called him the "engineer", not only because he held an engineering degree but also due to his rigidity and unyielding character. They told me that once he set his mind on something, nothing could sway him. Despite the nickname, he was highly regarded in the pavilion. Fortunately for

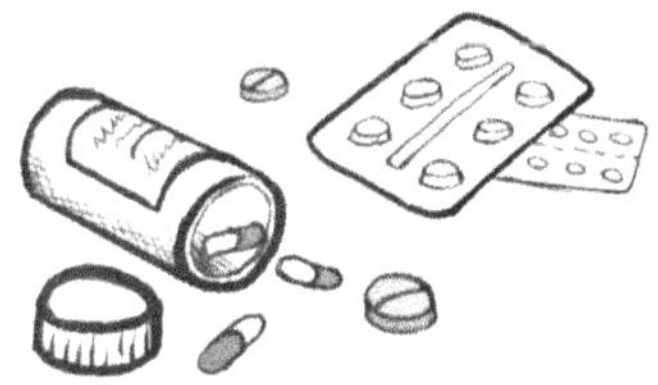

Fig. 5.3 Pills

him, his case had not attracted public attention; he was not one of the "well-known women killers" featured in the news. This allowed him to maintain a low profile in prison.

Héctor agreed to an initial interview, courtesy of his closest cellmate who introduced us. The interview would be, based on his proposal, a trial to test if he was comfortable with the situation. Should he feel uneasy about it, we would stop the interview and I would delete the recording.

Our meeting started on the right foot: he invited me for a coffee and the conversation started flowing. "It makes no sense that we beat around the bush, right? You came here to talk about Priscila, the missus." He started his story by telling me about the relationship he had with his wife, his "missus":

> We met at that time in life when everything was possible. I had just finished university, I was 24. I had finished my degree at a very young age, for engineering school. Even today, when the academic level has decreased acutely, people don't finish their course at 24. And she had just started working as a secretary in the firm I had joined, as an intern. Then I climbed my way up to a permanent position. [...]. We had a knock-out. The vultures at the office hovered around her, day and night. But I was the one who ended up with her in the end [smiles].

Héctor and Priscila started dating shortly after they met, in 1984. She was 18 years old and had just started working against the wishes of her father, who wanted her to become a primary teacher. However, she wanted to start working right away and become independent. "She was always a rebel", Héctor said.

Héctor was keen to talk about what he called the "honeymoon phase": their first year as a couple and their first years of marriage. This stage was, by his logic, the benchmark against which he compared the rest of their relationship:

> Going out to have a nice pulque [agave wine], travelling to the beach, taking her by surprise to have a nice coffee in the city centre. The first times were like that, as it should be, right? It's the moment to discover her, make her fall in love, smitten her. I was over the moon.

They dated for almost three years before he proposed. Before doing so, he asked for her father's permission: already at that time, this was seen as slightly old-fashioned. Without me asking him, Héctor felt the need to explain himself: "it seemed like the right thing to do, because my father-in-law had always been her moral compass."

> Tying the knot was an important moment. Getting married was at that time not a light affair like today. One does not simply go into a civil registry, with the idea that that union might dissolve at some point. It was a pact for the rest of your life. I believe we both joined the institution of marriage with this idea in mind. It was for like, having faith that we would build something ourselves.
> I bought our first house a few years after we got married. I had the financial opportunity to purchase it, as an engineer. She was no longer working, she was taking care of our home. And since we didn't have children at that time, we had a lot of spare time for ourselves, like we were still dating, right?
> A normal day was to wake up at six, have breakfast, go to the office until four or five, depending on the workload, and then get back at home and have a snack ready. We always went for a substantial snack rather than a heavy dinner.

In his meticulous descriptions of their daily routine, Héctor found a way to convey the idea of homely tranquillity. Building a story that accounted for this initial period of joy and stability served to accentuate the contrast with later periods of chaos and suffering. The differentiating of a before and an after was a structuring theme of our talks: whether it was regarding the academic standards of the universities, the way in which the people think about marriage or their relationship, the 'before' always shone on the prospects of the present.

Two years after getting married, they had their first child: Carlos. The arrival of his firstborn was a watershed moment for Héctor. Not only did this event a drastically change their home dynamics, his son monopolised Priscila, creating a gulf between her and Héctor:

> I know it's controversial to frame it like that, but Carlitos consumed her. Day and night she was there for him. Obviously, she was a new mother and it is logical that she would focus on her son. But it was unhealthy, let's say, that level of attachment. For example, she breastfed him until he was two years old. That… is not normal [laughs].
> I always said that something broke in the relationship at that moment. Actually, something broke in her then. Maybe her maternal instincts were too young, she wasn't ready, I don't know. Later I realised that there were other issues. Of her mental health. Deeper issues that she had been dragging, and that she continued dragging throughout her life.

In Héctor's story, the arrival of their son was a turning point in his relationship with Priscila and led him to gradually distance himself from her:

> The years went by and things got worse. I don't think I realised how bad she was until it was too late. That's why I feel… I feel very guilty. I am stricken by remorse to think that if I had realised her state earlier, things would have ended differently. But then I think: how could I have noticed? When I say that time passed, I mean that years, decades passed. We had a daughter later, when Carlitos was two years old. It was a great relief when she arrived, because she brought with her peace. It wasn't the three of us, inexperienced parents and a boy crying all day. We were two parents with more experience, a little older boy, and a beautiful girl who smiled all the time. I had a closer, more affectionate bond with her. To this day, she makes anyone smile. When Priscila was fifty years old, fifty eh, the bond was different. As one would expect in any relationship, right? We had been together for more than thirty years by that time, two kids, a grandson, a lifetime together. But that's where it started, which made me wake up and realise something was wrong. I even remember that

day! He says enthusiastically. She had come back from having tea with some neighbours and she told me that she wanted to go back to work. Betty, her friend, needed people in the administration of the school she ran and she suggested Priscila could take over that position. Now, think about this, my wife hadn't worked since she was twenty. What was she going to do there!? Makes no sense. And besides, she tells me that she was locked up all day, that she didn't know what to do, that she felt controlled, suffocated, she said. But that was when I began to realise it, when I began to suspect that something was wrong, that something was happening to her. I met with a lifelong friend, a psychiatrist, in a café. We met in high school and have been friends ever since. And I told him about the situation. From one day to the next, my woman started saying that she wanted to work, that she felt empty, that she didn't know what to do anymore, that she couldn't be locked up all day. Besides, she was never one to have many friends, right? So what did she expect? Of course she felt this way. But why not before? My friend begins to ask me more about her life, about her state of mind, mood swings, fights, day-to-day mood. I remember that he asked me how her days were organised. Sure, I have no idea about psychiatry, but he figured it out. She was depressed. De-pressed!

The moment Héctor 'realised' that Priscila suffered from a mental disorder was an epiphany that fundamentally reshaped his perception of her and their entire relationship. This revelation not only gave him a new framework for interpreting her behaviour but also influenced his actions moving forward. However, within the context of the abuse in their relationship, framing her situation as depression could also be seen as another form of avoidance and a means of exerting control over her.

In the background of his story, a recurring theme began to surface: Priscila's autonomy. Her parenting style, the way she managed household chores, her time spent having tea with friends, and, ultimately, her desire to return to work became central to Héctor's narrative, closely intertwined with his interpretation of her mental health.

Héctor came up with several possible strategies to address this perceived problem. However, talking to her was not an option: she would not come to her senses, she never had. Talking to the few friends she had was even worse: they would surely encourage her to work and take less care of herself. They were never to his liking. He did not want to include his children in the conversation: Carlitos was not going to understand that his perfect mother had a problem; Ludmila had other things to worry about:

> It was not an easy decision. After so many years together, one would think that it is easier to get to know the other person, their secrets, how to talk to them. But it's not like that. We are unpredictable. [...]. I opted for the best of all evils. Knowing that there were not many options, seeing her worse every day, I took the bull by the horns. I asked my friend to prescribe medication for her. The medication that he would give to a patient like her, in her condition and with that mental condition. He understood the delicate situation, being in a tight spot. And we launched into this covert operation.

The plan was, in its own way, straightforward. The psychiatrist—a trusted partner in this endeavour—would provide monthly prescriptions for lithium and, if required, risperidone. They also contemplated the potential use of amitriptyline. Although these medications belong to different families (lithium, a mood stabiliser; risperidone, an atypical antipsychotic; and amitriptyline, a tricyclic antidepressant), they all serve to regulate mood, emotions, and behaviour, making them key devices in controlling individuals. Héctor would crush the pills and discreetly mix them into her meals. In the short term, the aim was to calm her and alleviate her restlessness. In the long term, they hoped she would return to her usual self.

> And so we started. One Sunday, when I made breakfast, I put the powder in the yoghurt. Since she always cooked, I decided to start a less suspicious day. Then I just found any possible occasion. And that day she fell asleep right away. It was summer, so she thought it was heat stroke [laughs].

The strategy continued for four months. Héctor proudly shared with me the progress he had made over those months. Although she started working, she interpreted her constant tiredness as a sign of exhaustion and stress. Maybe it was not the right time to go back to work. Maybe Héctor was right.

Héctor' story reached a climax in which all the small details that he had previously mentioned converged: the change in their relationship, Priscila's mental health, the *status quo* and the coercive control strategies:

> And one day everything went to hell. I think she never suspected anything. I was always careful and she never noticed [smiles]. But one Tuesday, when I was putting the smashed pills in the yoghourt, she saw me. She asked me what it was and that's where the fight started. [...]. She didn't believe me that it was sweetener [laughs]. That was the day of the incident. She went crazy.

Héctor's tone shifted registers. The humorous way in which he recounted his feat turned serious and fatalistic:

> Instead of being reasonable, she started yelling one day. She was shouting that I drugged her and other nonsense. I tried to explain to her what had actually happened, but she started threatening me, calling me crazy. I tried to explain at first that I was doing something to help her, that she was not well. I remember giving her an example to help her remember: when we were younger, she had checked my agenda, my phone book, to see who I had in there. I caught her, and we argued. At that moment, I told her it was the same situation. And that's when it all exploded. I didn't want her to leave because she was not well. Imagine, in that state: depressed, unreasonable, crazy. She was not stable. [Silence]. And I used, well, I used the gun to make her stay. As a feint, to scare her. To keep her there. She was not in her right mind [laughs]. No one... I can't tell anyone about this. Nobody wants to understand it. Like in A Confederacy of Dunces. The book. All crazy. She was leaving; she had packed a little suitcase with some things, she actually had it packed from before. When she was about to leave, I looked for the weapon in my office, and I told her not to go, and I shot. It all happened so fast.

Héctor described that moment partly in despair, partly with humour. However, he did not mention any mistakes or erroneous decisions on his part. To some extent, he almost described the situation as inevitable; the sequence of events unfolding as if clockwork. When I asked him about his experience of that last fight, he stressed the lack of options to address her 'condition':

> I felt a rush, accelerated, because she was leaving, and I wouldn't have been able to help her. It was going to be too late. I felt angry that there was no other option. Because, what was I going to do? Stay crossed-armed? Hospitalise her? [...]. When I shot, everything collapsed. The walls toppled down. A weird feeling, like being between a rock and a hard place.

I felt his determination and despair as he spoke. I have listened to countless other men claim that they had 'no options', yet never so forcefully as Héctor. When I asked him about the gun, he brought up the confidentiality of the interview. It seemed that this issue, unlike the other topics we addressed, was more sensitive:

> I told you everything. I am not sure why you would need all this. I do not know how it could be of use. Yes, for your thesis. I do not disparage that type of work. I am, anyway, here [in prison].

Héctor asked me to stop recording our conversation. He had had enough. We met one more time to review the transcripts and agree on the main aspects he wanted to cover. I was also interested in knowing why he agreed to participate in the interviews. Unsurprisingly, he stressed that, while knowing this was an anonymous recording, he wanted to set the record straight: his relationship with Priscila was not a violent one; it was based on love. All his actions were intended to help her.

* * *

Coercive control frequently emerged as a prominent theme among the men interviewed, offering a crucial lens for understanding intimate partner violence more broadly. As an interpreter of their stories, one can subtly discern this issue in side notes or adjacent remarks; for some, it was woven into the fabric of their relationships. For Héctor, however, coercive control served as a defining element of his self-presentation. Maintaining dominion over Priscila was a central thread in his narrative:

whether it involved reproductive autonomy, economic abuse, or physical independence, control was fundamental to constructing a coherent story.

In Héctor's account, control was also woven as a remedial strategy to counter Priscila's autonomy, but more broadly, her desires. This narrative could, however, be interpreted in two ways. On one hand, it is a story illustrating how domination might restore balance in the face of perceived threats or fears (e.g., of loneliness or fragility). In this sense, control becomes an inherently performative act, a means to feel and identify as powerful—thus a way of "doing gender" (West & Zimmerman, 1987). Conversely, control might also be understood as a way to establish communion: a narrative emphasising how controlling behaviour enables connection. For Héctor, intimacy was only achievable through control.

This vignette also foreshadows other stories—explored in Chapter 6—that highlight the role of social relationships in both control and femicide. Héctor's strategic request for help from the psychiatrist friend—much like other men who turn to social resources—enabled him to navigate undetected, gain support, and sustain his coercion. Seeking assistance, whether from friends or colleagues, becomes a calculated move to reinforce control while maintaining a façade of legitimacy, often serving to deflect scrutiny or weaponise external systems to his advantage.

Beyond shedding light on the extreme forms of coercive control, Héctor's story also serves as a gateway to understanding avoidance. Forcing medication on Priscila without her knowledge, for instance, functioned as a strategy to conceal the very presence of control. For us, as readers and listeners of this story, it becomes a clear example of "leaking" (Rumpf et al., 2024): the unintended or subtle exposure of controlling behaviours or manipulation that are usually hidden or denied, often revealing the underlying dynamics of abuse within patterns of intimate terrorism.

While writing this vignette in 2024, the case of Gisèle Pélicot came to light, sparking international outrage as a harrowing example of sustained abuse. Her husband, Dominique Pélicot, was accused of orchestrating and facilitating her drugging and repeated rape over several years, often within their home in Mazan, France. This case, when juxtaposed with Héctor's narrative, invites critical reflection on the universality of coercive control across geographical, cultural, and social contexts. It raises significant questions: are these men more alike than different? Can such shared patterns redefine femicide as a singular, global phenomenon?

Telling the Stories of Policing, Emotions and Resources

Jorge, Celso, and Héctor exemplify what Kate Manne (2020) describes as "overachievers" of violence: individuals who enact misogyny with a degree of precision and intensity that surpasses others in their social contexts. Their relentless pursuit of controlling their intimate partners escalated to the point where it culminated in heinous murders. In this chapter, I have deliberately presented these cases in a manner that highlights the gender normative aspect of these femicides, to emphasise how central this attitude is to this kind of violence.

A striking aspect of these narratives is the element of policing of women. This can manifest itself in various forms, such as reproductive coercion, intimate terrorism, and unequal pay. These cases prominently feature infractions, punishment, and a sense of entitlement to impose sanctions. Rule-breaking indicates that, within a given social context, there are tacit rules that are accompanied by certain sanctions when they are violated. In these stories, all of these rules remained implicit. The men acted in response to perceived violations of an incontestable gender status quo, no matter how ridiculous or trivial these infractions may seem to us as readers.

These are not unfamiliar stories; we have encountered them in classical literature, films, TV dramas, and even memes. However, a common analytical misunderstanding, I believe, is the tendency to separate structural policing from the subjective mechanisms through which it is enacted. The stories I have heard are primarily about feelings of hurt, threat, and confusion—narratives in which men feel overwhelmed by a reality they perceive as unfair and impossible to control. Ultimately, these are embodied narratives (Di Marco & Sandberg, 2024). Both Jorge and Celso vividly describe the physical sensations they experienced during their conflicts, while Héctor illustrates how emotions, rather than reasoning, drove his actions. It is crucial to remind ourselves that, despite the dominant assumption that we are Cartesian beings, we are also deeply influenced by emotions inscribed in our bodies (Rosaldo, 1994).

Interpreting these stories as tied to gender regulation, yet as embodied norms, raises questions about the rules governing these emotions (Hochschild, 1979). Surveillance, rule-breaking, and the subsequent punishment can ultimately be seen as forms of *remediatory action*: the control exerted, and the final act of killing—regardless of intentionality—may be understood as compensatory for perceived emotional and moral damage (Fahs et al., 2023). From this lens, there is no issue with a lack of emotional literacy in these men. On the contrary, it is a matter of the literacy they (and we) already possess.

In my reading of these cases, it is key to consider the emotional and instrumental aspect of lethal violence, as it situates these actions within a material and symbolic context. Femicides are inevitably about controlling women, but they are also attempts to control 'resources'. These crimes are linked to a rupture over assets. Jorge attempted to exert control over his partner, making decisions about her body in an instrumental and domineering manner; Celso ruminated on trust as a scarce resource in intimate relationships; and Héctor asserted sovereignty over 'his housewife'.

It would be misleading to reduce misogyny to mere hostility or hatred towards women harboured by men. When confronted with this definition, one must ask: why? What is invested in these relationships that becomes so important? Misogyny is fundamentally about controlling and punishing women who challenge male dominance. This is why the logic of punishment operates so systematically: misogyny reinforces the status quo and punishes those who do not. This transactional approach helps us understand that misogyny is ultimately a social system "in which women will tend to face hostility of various kinds because they are women in a man's world (i.e., a patriarchy)" (Manne, 2017, p. 33).

Hopefully, it will become clear to the reader that stories are a central element in these cases. We do not only access this phenomenon through them—whether through the stories of the victims, the justice system, the media, or the activists—but these stories also serve as instigators of the crimes themselves. It is through these narratives that we, as people within the same system, denaturalise how we relate to one another.

6

Zooming Out

The three cases I presented in the previous chapter focus on the emotional and moral contours of intimate femicide. By highlighting feelings, experiences, and expectations, these vignettes illustrate some of the underlying logics of this form of harm doing (Fig. 6.1). These narratives, however, fall short in depicting the broader social contexts of the events: they are stories specifically constructed to centre on the man-woman dyad. Thus, a superficial interpretation of these vignettes could lead to a biographical illusion (Bourdieu, 2017), suggesting that femicide occurs independently of social contexts. This is not due to a lack of environmental descriptions, but rather because these contexts were not emphasised in the stories themselves.

Femicides do not occur in social isolation. They predominantly take place in urban spaces, surrounded by tight networks of relatives, friends, acquaintances, schools, healthcare facilities, and a multitude of other social actors. They also happen after a longer period of abuse, with potentially recognisable red flags. Men who commit this extreme form of violence are not akin to Robinson Crusoe—a myth based on the idea of societal ground zero—living on a deserted island without CCTV, colleagues, or families.

M. H. Di Marco, *Narratives of Femicide Perpetrators in Latin America*,
https://doi.org/10.1007/978-3-031-97367-3_6

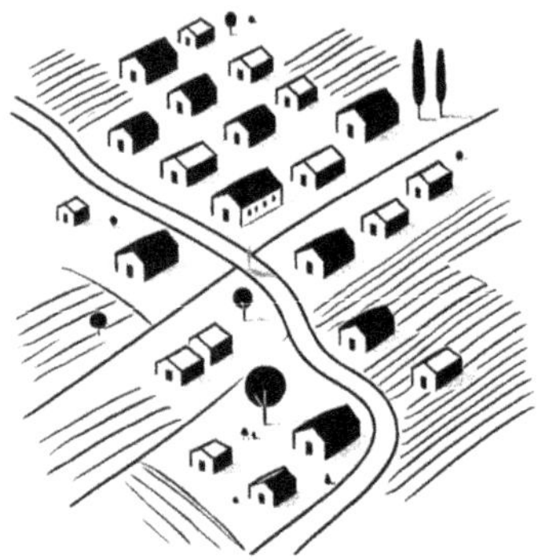

Fig. 6.1 Zooming out

This poses a conundrum for understanding these killings: Were there no bystanders? Did the social circle attempt to intervene? What roles do institutions play in these crimes? More importantly, from a narrative lens, I wonder: how are these networks perceived by the perpetrators? Are they seen as adversaries or allies in their narratives? Were their stories helpful in navigating institutions and 'flying under the radar' of the State prior to the crime?

In this section, I present three vignettes that provide a broader perspective on intimate femicide, bringing into focus the often-overlooked social contexts surrounding these crimes. These narratives expose the intricate web of actors, institutions, and environments that shape the conditions in which intimate femicides occur, demonstrating that these crimes involve more than just stories about women. Matías' story underscores the crucial role that friends can play in enabling male violence. João's account of his violent childhood and subsequent intimate relationship adds further context to the dynamics at play. Lastly, José's story reveals how these narratives can provide insight into the active role of institutions, such as the police, in their failure to intervene before the homicide occurred.

Matías: Male Brotherhood

> I understand, of course, that what we did was wrong. I'm not daft, nor am I a psychopath. I take responsibility for the mess I got us into, but who wouldn't do the same? Seriously, think about it. Your mate, your lifelong mate, messes up, hits someone – aren't you going to lend a hand? Are you going to say, "No, mate, we have to go to the police station"? Never in my life have I heard someone say or do something like that. In films, sure, we're all law-abiding citizens and whatnot. But in real life, we help our mates.

I met Matías through a friend of his. They had shared a prison cell for three years and became inseparable (Fig. 6.2). "He's a guy you can trust; he stands by your side", his friend told me. At the time, I did not realise just how important friendships were in Matías' story—how male peers had been there throughout his life, shaping key moments. The biggest lesson I took from my conversations with him was about the central role male friendships play. It is not just that male bonding and 'loyalties' reflect a broader, male-dominated society; they are actually crucial to its very reproduction.

In our first encounter, Matías was friendly and outgoing. He agreed to participate to get his story heard by others and 'show' how logical his actions were:

> I had a pretty normal life, I'd say. Until this moment, of course. But, you know, I grew up with both of my parents, attended school, had my

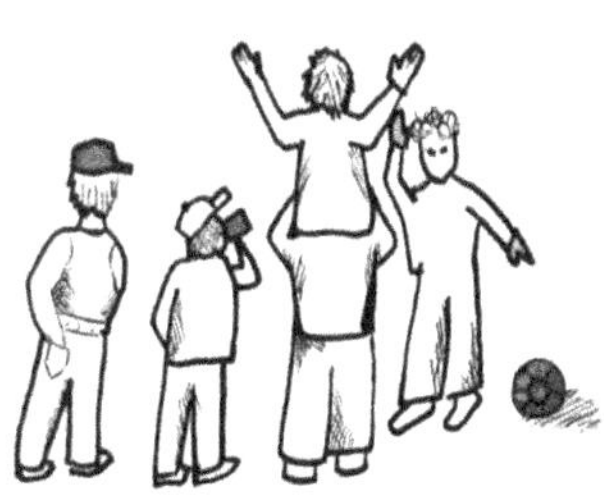

Fig. 6.2 Bro hood

> first job when I was 18, had my girlfriends, had my wife. I used to play football every Sunday. Nothing out of the ordinary. This was just… out of the blue, something that crashed me, but definitely this was not what I am.

Matías was born and raised in a middle-class family in the early 1960s. He was the eldest of three brothers. His father, a respected lawyer in the community, had his own firm. His mother was trained as a primary teacher and became a full-time homemaker when she had her first child. Matías depicted his childhood as filled with what he perceived as 'ordinary' activities and experiences. Even when he described how his father would be physically abusive, this was presented as unproblematic and part of a traditional and expected parental disciplinarian approach. "He would spank me and my brothers, but it was nothing violent, just good old-fashioned corrective measures."

When Matías turned 14, he had his first sexual experience with a woman. Sergio, his older cousin, took him to a sex work establishment in a nearby city. He described this place as "the poor version of my hometown. You could buy anything you needed there, if you had the money and the courage to go there":

> I guess that was more normal at that time. Now with feminism things are changing and it is frowned upon. But I think it is just normal: you are horny, inexperienced and young, so going to a prostitute seems like an obvious thing. And she gets paid; the oldest job in the world, right? [...]. And for me it was good, because I met my first girlfriend just that summer, so it was nice to have some experience.

This moment was not only a pivotal event in which he became 'closer to an adult', but also crucial in forging a stronger bond with his cousin:

> He was... I admired him so much. He was only one and a half years older than me, yet he seemed so worldly. He was knowledgeable and incredibly confident. He had a way of talking himself out of any situation, and the girls adored him! I believe he was actually my first true friend.

Curiously, while Matías described his visit to the establishment as his first sexual experience—or his "debut"—he later recounted how he used to masturbate with his friends. Reflecting on these sporadic and adventurous moments with his school friends, he laughed them off, saying, "It was just a fun childish thing to do."

Matías met Rosa just after he turned 15; she was still 13 at that time. They both attended the same school. She had just transferred there, since her family moved to that city. She was, as he describes, "unproblematic":

> I remember it like a nice relationship. Everything was quite new for both, and since she was basically new in town, there was not much problem dating her. You know, nobody had dated her before, she was not taken, no rumours, no nothing. She was unproblematic [giggles].

They dated for one and a half years, until the chemistry "stopped working" for them. In this mind, they both grew out of the love they felt. She was no longer the sweet and innocent girl he had once liked, and had become more interested in other things:

> At some point, I thought: what am I doing? She has other interests now, and it seems we are no longer a 'we'. Like, I was not willing to stop having a normal relationship, spending the time we used to spend together, because she was more interested in doing [school] extracurricular things. So, I ended it.

Playing football and hanging out with his friends kept him going. The pain of ending a relationship was eased by his close circle of friends, who distracted him and occasionally introduced him to other girls. During this period, Sergio played a significant role: he would pick him up after school for a beer or a game of pool. "In hindsight, I view my relationship with Sergio as magnetic. It was cyclical: some years we were inseparable, other years we were more distant. But we deeply cared for each other."

After completing high school, Matías began working in a bank. A close acquaintance of his family was the director of a local branch of a major regional bank and hired him for basic administrative tasks. Matías' world changed drastically: he was now economically independent, living on his own, and embarking on a new chapter in his life.

The following years passed uneventfully. The events that unfolded during those years were all considered expected. Matías skipped over several years of his life in his narrative: he did not describe his romantic relationships during that period, how his career progressed, his vacations, or his relationship with his family. These occurrences seemed insignificant compared to the next stage of his life.

When he was 25, Matías met María de los Ángeles. She was 20 at the time. They had a friend in common, who was celebrating their birthday. They met at a party on a Saturday evening. The attraction was immediate. He found her beautiful, but predicted a tragedy from the start:

> Matías: That type of woman is usually very conflictive. I mean, nothing so beautiful comes uncomplicatedly. And at the beginning it was great. But it would never work out.
> Martín: Why?
> Matías: She was too complicated, too unstable, too carefree. She was a beautiful crazy girl.

Matías and María de los Ángeles saw each other for three months, until she stopped it. She had decided to continue dating an ex-boyfriend. For Matías, those months happened fast. When I asked him about the relationship itself, he said it was a smooth and fun relationship. Since none of both actually had any serious interest, expectations were low, and there was no conflict.

Matías met his wife, Helena, by the end of that year. She worked in a shop near his office and had matched on Tinder. They got married two years after they started dating. During our conversations, he hardly talked about her. She was less of an active person in his daily life, and more of a supporting character of his narrative. The daily struggle of his job, football anecdotes and politics were more mentioned than his relationship with her.

Three years after the wedding, Matías's life seemed stable on the surface, but his story began to reflect growing dissatisfaction with his daily routine and his relationship.

> One day, I ran into her [María de los Ángeles] on the street. I hadn't seen her in quite a while; we chatted and decided to have something to drink. And what happened? We felt that spark again. That's when we started seeing each other again.

Matías and María de los Ángeles started having an affair. Matías described it as an adventure, with excitement and joy. There was nothing morally conflicted about the situation: it was more a question of dodging potential risks, being caught, and not letting it interfere in his 'normal' life. Yet the relationship changed one day when María de los Ángeles told him she was pregnant:

> It was as though she had poured a bucket of cold water over me. She said, "I'm pregnant," and the first thing that came to my mind was that I would lose everything. I would lose my wife, I would lose a divorce case, I would lose my job. I imagined a catastrophe [...]. I couldn't envision a future without everything going to shit.

Matías described going through a tremendous meltdown. Not only was this moment pivotal (it changed how he saw her, his life, and his actions), but it impacted what he would do in the near future. He asked her to have an abortion. She had already thought about this and, while this was not legal, it was a common and extended practice in the country. He decided that the best and safest option was to call his cousin. He was now a physician, working in the public health care system, and would certainly know what steps to follow:

> Two days later, she was heading to the primary healthcare facility. She had it. My saviour [cousin] helped me, and everything went smoothly. At that time, I thought, 'Phew, I dodged the bullet.'

As his wife, María de los Ángeles was never an active participant in the decision-making process; she was the complicated aspect of the equation. Matías perceived a conflict that, in his narrative, seemed to stem from external forces. It was his strong bond with his cousin that served as the touchstone through which the issue was resolved.

Matías described the abortion, or more accurately his convincing her to have one, as a triumph. As he told me, it was "going back to the path of sanity". However, María de los Ángeles disagreed. She endured the situation, feeling deeply affected by it. Intense discussions followed over the next two weeks: she realised his actions had overstepped her boundaries and felt used. The final conversation was in her house:

> She kept insisting, "You used me," but I argued that she was equally responsible for everything. "I never forced you to do anything," I told her, but she was hysterical. Then she threatened, "I will tell your wife. This won't be kept just between us."

The threat of telling his wife about the affair and the abortion was a breaking point for him. He described that moment as feeling not only aghast but terrorised. This shattered his bubble: he imagined being abandoned by his wife, his family finding out, and his colleagues thinking he was a cheater. That was not part of his plans.

In the next fifteen minutes of the interview, he described the femicide. He explained that her mention of telling someone about their affair was a trigger. He slapped her and then began hitting her with closed fists until he lost control of his actions. For him, it was important to convey that he did not plan the homicide. It was an action grounded in the "heat of the moment":

> I called my cousin. If there was anyone I could trust about this, it was him. I guess we all have someone who we can trust even for the worst. He drove there and was in the same state of shock as me. I remember he tried to calm me down, saying that it was not my fault, that she had used psychological violence on me and that the abortion was also strenuous to me.

Matías and his cousin attempted to move her body. Their plan was to drive to the countryside, find a secluded field, and dig a grave. Yet they did not expect that the fight called the attention of a neighbour, who called the police. They were caught in flagrante still in her house.

* * *

Matías's story contains several noteworthy elements, with the portrayal of men being particularly striking. He frequently referred to his male friends as pivotal figures in his life, recounted homoerotic experiences that were recast as fraternal adventures, justified his father's violent behaviour, and detailed his cousin's active role in the femicide. Together, these aspects underscore a prominent theme of male camaraderie throughout his narrative.

Homosociality—a concept originally coined by Eve Kosofsky Sedgwick (1985) and later expanded for instance by masculinity scholars like Michael Flood (2007) —not only highlights how men's bonds with each other shape their relationships with women but also actively influences them. Building on this idea, Whynacht (2017) argues that homosociality reveals how much of the violence experienced by women and non-conforming genders is ultimately mediated through men's social relationships with other men. In Matías' case, this support transcends the usual conceptualisation and denotes a much blunter meaning of male support.

As with all life story interviews, maintaining vigilance against biographical illusion is crucial. In Matías's case, his storytelling focused on presenting himself as a heterosexual man despite engaging in homoerotic practices. It also involved framing his affection and loyalty to his cousin as a macho alliance, describing their relationship as "magnetic". This presentation echoes other interviews where male friendships play pivotal roles (acting as watershed moments in life stories), yet are often portrayed with stoicism. Whether this can be understood as condensing and displacing (Lacan, 1973) emotions like love, or as the practice of silencing, enabling, and complicity among friends in intimate partner violence (DeKeseredy & Schwartz, 2013), these elements in the narratives can easily go unnoticed if the story is accepted at face value.

One small revelation I only noticed months later, while reviewing the transcripts, was that the interviewees I used to construct Matías' vignette never mentioned their wives by name. Instead, these men referred to them using terms like "my wife", "her", or simply ellipses, which emphasised their role rather than their subjectivity as independent individuals. In contrast, friends and cousins played a much more prominent role in how they presented themselves.

Matías' story, and my aim in presenting this biographical composite, is to spark a conversation about the broader context of femicide and, more specifically, how male bonds contribute to various forms of gender-based violence. Brotherhood—and its many conceptualisations in academia—ultimately highlights the conditions that make such violence possible. In my view, this extends beyond intimate partner femicide and is a fundamental condition for how conflicts are handled and emotions are processed in many, particularly Western, societies.

João: Hushed Neighbourhoods

"That old woman next door looked me in the eyes. She had the most intense piercing glance. But I knew she was not going to make a fuss." Silencing and secrets were the linchpin of João's story (Fig. 6.3). They were not only an element that made his story organic, which would otherwise be incoherent, but also a resource mobilised to make the story happen.

João was 41 years old when I interviewed him. He was raised in the countryside of a big city. He described the small town of 2000 inhabitants as desolate, with the crumbling facades of buildings after waves of recession and economic crisis. From the story he told, I could decipher what people did in this place: he sometimes referred to the agrarian activities of the province, the tractors going by, and the long history of farming and trained ranchers. Yet his parents had always been unemployed. They made a living out of state support and occasionally small on-the-side jobs, like mowing lawns.

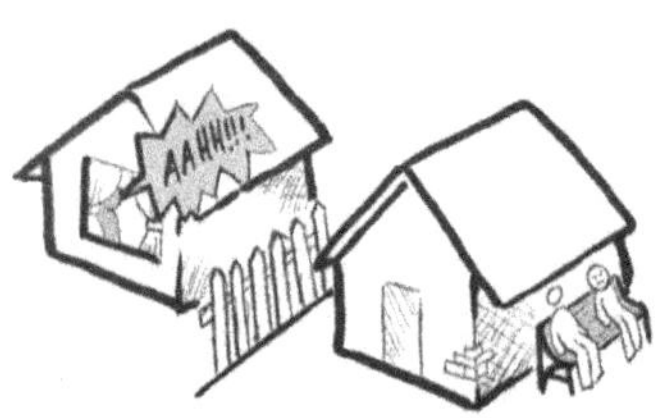

Fig. 6.3 Neighbourhood

João grew up with seven siblings, and two half-siblings. His childhood home was the centre of parties and meetings, and it was also the beginning of João's use of cocaine:

> My house started... It was a gathering place. A bunch of kids, friends of my brother and sister, used to come over. And that's when I started using drugs [marijuana and cocaine] secretly with them. I started drinking alcohol and I didn't want to be at home anymore. I started meeting other people who stayed on the street. Nothing. I left. I mean, I went downtown. Like, I would go downtown and return home after a few days. And when I went home, it was, I don't know, to check on my sister, and I remember bringing her a bunch of stuff. I mean, I remember feeling better when I was on the street. When I was at home, sometimes I didn't even eat, and when I was on the street, I was better than when I was at home. That's why I... And I would go home and have nothing to eat, so I would bring stuff.

I found it difficult to have a clear notion of João's zigzagging living trajectory. Sometimes he described spending months living in the streets and being completely estranged from his relatives, yet he would later describe having a mate on a rainy Sunday afternoon with his mother. The relationship became clearer when he started talking about his father's moodiness:

> Because when he would get those attacks he was very frightening. We wouldn't know if it was a bad day, an ok day, or the last day at all. I tried to avoid him as much as possible. Learned a lot about how to evade him. My siblings as well. Actually, the four eldest ones had already left by that point.

I interpreted that the ebb and flow of moving to the street and returning home were closely tied to the cycles of aggression from his father. Unlike other stories, where institutions like school serve as an organising force in their lives, his narrative centred around avoiding conflicts with his father as the primary strategy. It also became evident that the geography of the small town played a pivotal role in his story: the desolate nature of the town, its deserted streets, and the palpable depression brought on by waves of economic recession created the perfect environment for the father's violence to go unnoticed by the neighbours:

> That Saturday at 2 PM, the streets were empty. Everyone was taking a nap, and there was no way anyone could hear my dad's yelling. When he threw the tray at my mom and it hit the fridge, only the dogs were barking. The neighbour's German Shepherd knew more about what was going on than the neighbour did.

João moved out of the house when he was 15. Considering himself an adult at that age, he dropped out of high school as soon as he had enough money to make ends meet. He began taking on minor informal jobs in the town centre. He worked as a dishwasher for six months, then took an evening job at a kiosk. When he turned 16, he started working at a petrol station. Although it was illegal for him to work there, he made an agreement with the owner: he would receive no social benefits or social security and only work night shifts, where there were no controls.

During those years, he continued using marijuana and cocaine on a regular basis. His use was, in his words, "contained". He compared himself to other boys from his neighbourhood who had been using *merla*—a highly addictive, cheap, highly toxic form of crack cocaine, made from unrefined cocaine paste mixed with solvents—for over five years. In contrast, he only used it on weekends and believed it had no impact on his daily life.

When João turned 18, he secured formal employment at the petrol station. This was a significant milestone for him: being formally employed under a contract not only meant a stable income but also legal protection in case of a workplace accident. Having heard numerous stories from his friends, workplace accidents were seen as a spectre haunting those entering the job market.

Until that point, João had not mentioned dating or having sex. However, things were different at that point. He was not just an adult man; he was already thinking about settling down. His parents had started their relationship when they were both 19. His eldest brother had his first child at 17, and his elder sisters became mothers at 18 and 19.

Therefore, becoming a proper 'adult man' made sense within the context of his story:

> I felt it was time, you know? To stop fooling around and get more serious. I could keep messing around, but I was already thinking about my mates, who had kids, and I was like, "Hey, I want this too."

That was the preamble João shared before describing how he met Juliana. She was hired as a petrol station attendant to work the evening shifts. At the time, João was 19 and she had just turned 18. However, they did not hit it off right away. She was in a relationship when they met, and despite his attempts to court her, she resisted:

> She was playing hard to get. She'd say no, that she didn't want to because she had a boyfriend, but she kept trying to sweet-talk me all the time [laughs]. She'd come in all dolled up, wearing tight leggings, and you could see her thong [smiles]. I played it cool for a while, but about four months later, they broke up and that's when we started hooking up.

João and Juliana dated for several months before moving in together. She moved into the small house he was renting on the outskirts of town. I had done fieldwork for several months in this place years before. João showed me some pictures of the house: the neighbourhood was also visible in the background. It seemed a tightly packed neighbourhood, houses lean against each other, their weathered walls barely a breath apart. Windows, often no more than rough openings covered with sheets or makeshift shutters, directly face those of the adjacent homes, offering an unfiltered view into each other's lives. The proximity seemed asphyxiating, where privacy was not only a luxury, but unfamiliar altogether.

Now, they shared the same job, schedule, and commute. They even started having the same group of friends, as his next-door neighbour and dealer would frequently invite them to parties:

> Leandro would invite us to a party at his place every now and then. It was a small town and we all knew each other, but we had a great time there. We would jump the hedge and be there on time. There was booze

> and dancing until the early hours. I think we went every week back then. We'd count down the days until we could go and have a blast.

Over the next year, their relationship continued, and with it, João described a gradual social isolation for both of them. As they started using more drugs, the night shifts, the lack of alternative social groups, and the daily monotony and tedium of the town became, in his words, unbearable:

> The night shifts were a bloody nightmare because we were knackered the next day. We never got much sleep, were in a foul mood, and knackered, so we started blowing all our money on weed. It was only natural that we started arguing. We were in a right strop all day long.

Up until that moment, João only described having occasional quarrels. "As long as we had a stash, we were good", said laughing. The first explicit description of a conflict in their relationship occurred when Juliana received a phone call from her ex:

> We were inside the petrol station. I saw her discreetly pick up the phone and go outside. I obviously realised someone was calling her. She left, and I went after her a couple of minutes later. When she hung up, I asked her about it. She tried to cover it up for a while, but then she confessed.

In our conversation, he omitted the reason why Juliana and her ex-partner talked; he did not mention any specific suspicion, fear, or event, just took for granted the wrongfulness of her action. Hence, he felt no need to justify his response. He said he slapped her hard and, after yelling, calmed down and went back inside.

Over the next four months, the violence escalated: he remembered becoming impulsive, irascible, and exasperated every time she grabbed her phone. At one point, she went to the police station after one of their confrontations where he hit her, but she did not end up filing a complaint. "In a place this small, filing a complaint is pointless. We all know each other. Everyone knows what happens in each house. Gosh, I hear every neighbour when they flush their toilet. But they do nothing, because it's a small town." However, three weeks later Juliana did file a complaint, and shortly after that, João had a restraining order issued against him, although he was not given an ankle bracelet. "There were no resources in the municipality, apparently."

João was forced to take a leave of absence from work. The owner suggested it would be the appropriate course of action until the situation cleared up. However, he had other plans. On a Friday evening, when João was confident she would be home after her shift, he dragged a 20-litre can of kerosene and set fire to the cottage. He fled the scene but was soon captured by the police two hours later on the main road crossing through the town.

* * *

In 1973, Ana Mendieta, a Cuban American artist, created the *Moffitt Building Piece*, a series of images depicting a common street pavement with a door from which blood dripped. The neighbourhood had recently experienced the killings of women. Drawing on the experimental and performative approaches of the 1960s and 1970s—similar to Garfinkel's breaching experiments (1967)—her aim was to observe and document the reactions of ordinary people to this scene. She captures how individuals walked by, noticed the bloodshed, and continued on their way without intervening. She accurately and graphically showed how people looked the other way.

A narrative exploration of a life story reveals how experiences are reconstructed from the present. Narration highlights which actors are mentioned, what events are thematised, and which narratives are accessible from today's perspective. João reconstructs a story of social isolation and desolation, with few protagonists in his story. Initially, his family played a central role but later faded from the narrative entirely. In his adult life, the owner of the petrol station and Juliana emerged as important recurring characters. Yet, a seemingly overlooked actor cannot be ignored: the neighbours. João and Juliana lived in one of the most densely populated areas of the district, where silence is not a common resource. However, similar to his parents, there was a notable absence of intervention from others in their conflicts.

Silencing, as Presser (2022) argues, is a powerful practice that conceals underlying power structures. It is an active practice, requiring individuals to ignore, dismiss, or essentially 'look the other way' in certain situations (Zerubavel, 2018). By interrogating and contesting these silences, we can begin to dismantle the power structures that both create and arise from what often goes unspoken. This narrative of muted neighbourhoods—essentially a functional reproduction against complaint—reflects a pedagogy of witness that aligns with this theorisation of silencing. However, we hardly know anything about the neighbours involved.

This raises important questions about interpretation. The story can be understood in two primary ways. One approach is through a realist life history lens, examining the actions or omissions of neighbours in intervening, disrupting, or engaging in any way. Alternatively, we can interpret the latent impunity present in the narrative—not only regarding actions he expected to go unpunished but also reflecting a symbolic trust in the local social fabric. João's omission of potential neighbourly responses may be indicative of a broader reliance on silencing. I turn to João's story to interpret the impunity with which he potentially acted, and, more certainly, with which he recounted his narrative. Yet I wish to exercise caution in this interpretation: the reliance on silencing and the sense of impunity lie more in the act of narrating the story now than in the events being recounted.

João's life story highlights the crucial role that social networks play in the enactment of violence. His narrative describes how relatives, neighbours, and friends failed to intervene in his adverse experiences as a child—specifically, his father's abuse—or in his own abusive behaviour towards his partner. However, the story itself, along with the apparent lack of resistance he encountered, reveals more about the tellable narratives, entitlement, and the permissions granted to him than anything else.

José: Blind Institutions

José presented himself proudly as a police officer. “I come from a family of police officers, and we will always have uniforms in our souls.” I interviewed him when he was turning 45 years old, and just after he had served five years of his 22-year sentence (Fig. 6.4). He was living in a special unit, designed specifically for prisoners who might be at risk of internal conflicts: usually police officers, military personnel, or even those convicted of human rights violations:

> I am here because I killed my ex-wife. It was classified as a femicide, but things are more complicated than people realise. You hear, “He killed his ex. He must be a monster,” and so on. But after years of a tumultuous relationship, back and forth over custody of the children, and strenuous circumstances, the reality is different. Oh, and people just love to learn that I am a cop. It is like I fit what they expect from “a killer”.

Like many other interviewees, he tried to portray his childhood as normal. He talked about his parents’ unity, their economic stability, and his admiration for his father. Highlighting these events from his early years was a crucial signpost for understanding his later story.

> I had the childhood every child should have. Both of my parents were together and relatively happy. My father was in the forces; he retired just a couple of years ago. My mother was a housewife and raised me and my three siblings, two boys and two girls. We owned our home; we never had to rent. [...]. In my family, for instance, I admired my dad because, as I said, he had a good job and went to work every single day. Every day, for

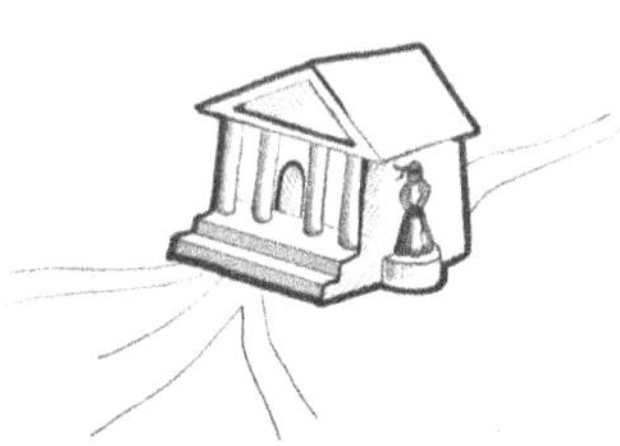

Fig. 6.4 Blind institutions

> example, he'd take a bath, always dressed in a uniform. I always thought I wanted to be just like him. I wanted to take a bath every day, dress up in a uniform for work, and earn a decent amount of money too. As I said, he even got paid when, well, you know, it wasn't always possible.

In some stories, the transition from childhood to adolescence was marked by the awakening of sexual desire; in others, it was the striving for independence from parents or starting to work. In José's case, it was primarily marked by his outspoken attempts to emulate his father's footsteps. For him, becoming a man meant transforming into a strong, stoic individual, taking charge of his life and becoming "confident", as he phrased it.

During his adolescence, the pursuit of becoming a robust man became his unspoken life project. He recalled taking sports very seriously, as "physical discipline is a foundational skill for developing a solid and controlled character". Studies were also included into this endeavour: "as people without any knowledge end up being pushovers or basically they always need others, they can't be actually independent if you are asking for advice all the time."

At a summer pool party, he met Abril. Both were in their mid-teens. She was the daughter of a local doctor. "Blonde, educated, responsible, sensual, yet still possessing street smarts", he described her. However, their relationship endured only for the season. His recounting of their courtship oscillated between being overwhelmingly attracted to her and perceiving her as unattainable:

> I was simply in awe. She was magnificent: everything she did, she excelled in – school, the summer fête she organised, her friends. I ought to have known she wasn't someone to hold onto; she was too beautiful, too perfect. By the end of that summer, I found myself cast aside.

As soon as he turned eighteen and completed high school, José joined the police academy. His entry into this new chapter differed significantly from that of most of his classmates: he had connections and an intimate understanding of the inner workings of the police force. Having met many of the instructors and staff at the training centre during his childhood, navigating his education was a smooth process. He completed the required courses on time, excelled in several of them, and promptly graduated at the top of his class.

From this moment onwards, José dedicated much of our conversations to describing his work in the police force. He detailed his training, highlighted how the police workforces had negatively changed compared to previous generations, and shared the daily chores and routines of his job. Being a policeman was perhaps the most defining aspect of his biography, a topic he repeatedly revisited to explain himself.

Years later, he encountered a young woman in a club. He was 29 and she was 23. It was a sweltering summer evening; the muggy December air was stifling on the crowded dance floor, so he stepped outside to share a beer with a police friend. It was there that he spotted Florencia passing by. He whispered, "You're a work of art in motion, babe". He referred to this as a "*piropo*" (pick up line), though I would prefer to call it catcalling:

> She was the kind of woman you only dream of. Truly a work of art, and with a very dark sense of humour. How could I let it pass? She was a gem. I made it my life's purpose to get her to marry me. Promised myself that that night.

They started dating after that night. José described their early relationship as a conquest: she was a goal to achieve, yet also symbolising an implicit asymmetrical dynamic. "She knew she was far superior to me, so I had to play the role of a warrior." However, his belligerent metaphor was more nuanced than I initially anticipated. Abril was not merely a conquest; she became the main focus amidst several 'sidequests'. Dating and engaging in intimate relationships with other women had been a habit he continued from the beginning of his relationship with Abril onwards:

> We all have a little something going on here or there. That doesn't distract you, or it shouldn't, from your real life. Your wife, your kids, your responsibilities. But if you feel the need, what can you do?

Abril and José married three years after that hot summer night, and two years after moving in together. Their marriage followed an heteronormative, archetypal trajectory: initial passion, followed by a perceived need to have children, the birth of Romina, and then settling into a phase of tedium and tension. José described this progression in a detached, almost monotonous manner. His reflections largely echoed conventional views and expressions about marriage, as if trying to underline the 'obviousness' of the situation or to forge a common understanding with me.

Romina was born during the early stages of the marriage. José introduced me to her during a videocall in one of our meetings. "She is the light of my eyes, everything I have in my life, and the reason I keep going, keep fighting", he said, smiling as he spoke.

After 12 years together, Abril filed for divorce, which did not surprise José. It was the culmination of two years of arguments over his numerous affairs. "The situation was unbearable", he said. "All day long it was nagging and chaos. It brought me down, so how could I not be with others?" José claimed her constant nagging and distress were actually signs of her wanting to end their marriage, interpreting them as expressions of boredom with their relationship:

> The breaking point, the moment when everything boiled over, was when we started discussing custody. Romina was... 8, no, 9 years old. And my ex-wife wanted to take custody away from me. She claimed I was a bad influence because I was a policeman, that I was violent, and that I had a gun. Of course! I'm in the force. That day, that argument, was the breaking point.

The custody battle was an intense period of conflict in his story. He had assumed the divorce would only cause minor changes, like "taking care of the house's legal scripts and scheduling Romina's days of the week," but he had not anticipated the chaos it became: "I did not sign up for the mayhem it turned out to be." The actual trial proved to be very different. Abril filed for full custody of their child, and José, in a deliberate attempt to damage her image, built a case in which he constantly belittled his ex-wife's ability to parent, insisting she was too emotional and unstable to care for their child:

> This was the moment I had to get resourceful. I reached out to a colleague who works with the municipal justice secretary for help. By then, I had been on the force for twenty years and knew the ins and outs of the municipality. My friends told me who to talk to, what to say, and what not to say. They even guided me on the timing. Without their help, I would have lost her, because usually, the women win these battles.

José was very clear about three things. First, he needed to acquire the know-how to understand and operate in the system. Second, he felt confident in contacting people, moving resources, and generally navigating the heavily bureaucratised gears of justice. Finally, he trusted that his friends and colleagues would believe his story, that it was convincing enough to mobilise his social capital, and that his actions were reasonable enough not to be hidden.

As the months of the judicial battle progressed, the conflict between them intensified. During this time, Romina spent the first four days of the week with her mother, then went to José's new apartment in the town centre. Since the streets were not safe enough for her to commute alone, José would pick her up. These moments often escalated into direct conflicts with Abril, and José admitted that, in some cases, he would yell and, "in the heat of the moment, take it out on a trash can."

> She filed for a restraining order. And, you know, I understand this world, I know how things work. Often, these orders are a tactic to scare off a man with a temper, not necessarily someone dangerous. Other times, it's a malicious attempt to weaken a father's bond with his children. It's women's rights gone wrong, tilted in their favour. It's pure injustice.

He saw the restraining order as a direct declaration of war. She was trying to retaliate against him for his infidelities by "taking away" their child. Two days after receiving the order, he called his closest friend, who had been a chief police officer in the municipality for three years:

> He knew Abril well; he knew she would be vindictive, and it wasn't out of fear. Regardless of our relationship, I would never harm my child. [...]. Apparently, there were some missing papers, her lawyer was not organised, and my friend managed to pull some strings. They annulled the restraining order.

José's story was unclear about the timing of events, with some parts seeming more spaced out than others. However, he emphasised that only two days passed between being notified about the order and successfully getting it annulled. He did not present this story as a proud accomplishment or a resourceful unfolding of events; to him, it was just an obvious consequence of the situation. "I did what any father would do in this situation. I picked up the phone and moved some contacts", he said.

José never talked about the femicide itself. From our conversations, I gathered that it happened just after he resumed contact with Abril. Like some other men, discussing the killing was off-limits for him. He was blunt about his lack of interest in discussing it with me:

> What happened later was a tragic accident. It was the result of exhausting circumstances: I was worn out from a long legal battle, just off a shift with my regiment, and dealing with her webs of lies and manipulations. I don't want to discuss it further; the press has already said enough.

Those words were from our last interview. However, I continued to meet José over the following months during my fieldwork at the prison. We regularly greeted each other and occasionally shared a drink in the courtyard. In his special unit, there was no shame about the femicide. He moved freely and almost unapologetically among other police officers, who, like his friends, supported his story.

* * *

José's story stands out for two main reasons: it is the story of a police officer, and it directly addresses how narratives can be used to navigate institutions or, in this case, circumvent norms. The fact that these two elements are brought up in one case is not random. Because of his position as a police officer, with a family background in that same institution, he managed to mobilise the contacts necessary to annul the restraining order.

Despite his apparent dexterity in navigating the judicial system, his story does not seem extraordinary or unusual. Considering how many femicides are perpetrated by police officers or military men worldwide (UNODC & UN Women, 2024), his story is rather exemplary of a broader pattern of perceived impunity and corruption. His story tells of a man who confidently asked for the assistance of his colleagues; the same protagonist who felt unapologetic about a victim-blaming narrative told in prison; and the same one who moved around the special unit without apparent remorse.

José's case can be interpreted from various perspectives. It can be viewed as a trajectory through institutional relationships or as an example of bureaucratic negligence. It can also serve as a proxy for silent institutional de-securitisation of intimate partner violence. Additionally, it could illustrate how individuals can leverage narratives to mobilise resources. Like João's case, José's story highlights the necessary silence that enables intimate femicide. José's account highlights the permeability of institutions and the stories that unlock these processes. Law enforcement and the justice system are depicted as malleable for individuals in his position. The avoidance, navigation, and strategic use of these institutions, along with the apparent reluctance of bureaucracies to intervene in 'private matters', emerge as prominent features of this case.

However, an underlying aspect of this self-presentation is how the self is perceived. This narrative can easily be mistaken for one of stoicism and a position of righteous power, as he frequently presents himself as resourceful and in control of the situation. Yet, I interpret it as a story of fragility, a weakened self, and a deep-seated fear of abandonment, along with an identification with a similarly fragile persona—his father. At a narrative level, turning to his peers and institutional support is, in essence, a declaration of impotence. José's vignette, like many others, serves as a cautionary tale about the illusions in self-presentation and the profound emotional turmoil underlying the stories they tell. Ultimately, his story is an attempt to compensate for the very feelings of impotence he strives to suppress.

Narrative Complicities

This chapter brings to the forefront the pivotal role of narratives about social relationships, contexts, and institutions. At its core, it resonates with a longstanding theoretical discussion on the interconnectedness between actions, beliefs, and contexts. In *A Contribution to the Critique of Political Economy* (1977 [1859]), Karl Marx famously critiqued the prevalent use of Robinsonisms—the idea of a societal 'ground zero' where an individual is depicted as self-sufficient and independent, much like Robinson Crusoe on his deserted island. This concept challenges lay and social theories that overlook or ignore the social conditions and collective interactions shaping individual behaviour and societal structures. Marx's critique addressed the widespread assumption of individual autonomy and highlighted that no one operates in isolation; rather, we are embedded in a complex web of social relationships and structures.

Despite Marx's critique nearly two centuries ago, and decades of vigorous feminist movilisation, contemporary discourse still risks perpetuating this same myth. Interpersonal violence is often analysed without considering its contextual or historical dimensions, crime is frequently understood in isolation from the biographies or meanings behind it, and homicides are commonly described without reference to the narrative reality in which they occur. Moreover, femicides are often detached from the institutional networks in which they unfold.

Matías, João, and José each wove into their narratives the presence or absence of friends, neighbours, colleagues, and public institutions. Their stories illustrate how these crimes are committed not only within the context of intimate relationships but also within a broader social fabric. The actions and rationales of these other actors were present and, in various ways, influenced the events. However, as I argued before, we must be cautious in interpreting the contexts described by these men. Primarily, I approach this context from a discursive perspective: they are presenting narratives about their interactions with friends, neighbours, and the social system they navigated. Thus, my focus is on how their descriptions of contexts and people are articulated and how these narratives shape our understanding of the broader social influences at play.

The first story highlights how the trust and support of male peers—or 'male brotherhood' and homosociality—can have a decisive impact on the lives of women. Male bonding plays a crucial role in perpetuating sexist attitudes (Flood, 2007). Naturally, this male brotherhood may be emphasised by the narrators to exaggerate the role of friends or to present a more stable support network than actually existed. Nevertheless, the story centres—whether in realist terms or as part of their narrative framing—on the role that friends played. In the context of the interviews, bringing to life the voices and support of their friends was important to them.

In the second story, the neighbourhood becomes significant as the setting where a femicide can occur. This narrative can be interpreted as a tale of impunity through isolation, reflecting a sense of entitlement and a belief that the perpetrators' actions would face no interference. This is illustrated by a taken-for-granted assumption (Zerubavel, 2018): the fear of 'interference' was not even mentioned in the story.

Finally, the last story zeroes in on a critical point: a police perpetrator. This narrative underscores the role of stories in navigating systems and prompts us to consider institutional responsibilities and the accountability of state agencies. It highlights how sexist attitudes permeate entrenched patriarchal institutions, such as the police (Whynacht, 2021). It is not surprising that so many femicides are committed by police officers.

When listening to these stories, I found it useful to consider the conditions that enable femicides as analogous to human trafficking. Walby (2024), for instance, makes it abundantly clear that for this crime to occur, a web of actors must act in concert. Local police must turn a blind eye, judges must halt investigations, and border controls should remain silent. While some may interpret this dynamic as indicative of eroding social cohesion or weak institutions, I argue that this perspective is rather Eurocentric, particularly regarding Latin American states that have struggled to establish themselves under challenging geopolitical conditions. Framing intimate femicides as products of a web of complicity shifts the focus away from the victim-perpetrator dyad. Since many of these murders have a prior history of abuse, the questions of prior alerts, interventions, and warning signs become paramount.

The stories in this chapter illustrate the roles of collegiality and support. On one hand, both formal and informal cultures obscure complaints (Ahmed, 2021). On the other, these silences alert us to an ongoing pedagogy of cruelty. As Segato (2016) argues, the repetition of violence normalises a landscape of cruelty and, in doing so, fosters low thresholds of empathy among people, which are essential for predatory behaviour. Routine cruelty is directly proportional to forms of narcissistic and consumerist enjoyment and the isolation of citizens through their desensitisation to the suffering of others.

Social support and silencing form the backbone of these narratives. The web of complicities is extensive, encompassing actors ranging from male friends and relatives to corrupt police institutions, as well as narratives that trigger support and justify complicity (regarding loyalty, unnecessary interventions, and the normalcy of intimate partner violence). This support was often taken for granted in the interviews; there is no need to defend or justify an interaction with neighbours or a bruise seen at the local healthcare clinic. It reflects what we might assume as trust, alliance, and organisational male power (Hearn et al., 2025).

Regardless of the factual accuracy of these relationships, these stories indicate the narratives that are available to men and deemed valid to tell. I hypothesise that, despite the tailored nature of these stories—intertwined with denials and discursive strategies—they illustrate what is considered legitimate behaviour and what is not. I would argue that these narratives provide a valid, albeit indirect, means of understanding the webs of complicity at play. Through them, we can gain insights into the actors and institutions involved.

7

Weather Vanes

> When you are in the middle of a story it isn't a story at all, but only a confusion; a dark roaring, a blindness, a wreckage of shattered glass and splintered wood... It's only afterwards that it becomes anything like a story at all. (Atwood, 1996, p. 330)

The social context plays a crucial role in understanding violence (Fig. 7.1). The discursive landscape shapes actions and determines what is regarded as moral or immoral, justifiable or unjustifiable, distinguishing harm from violence (Presser, 2013). Moreover, it provides individuals with the necessary framework to interpret their own behaviour and construct their sense of identity. In this way, the social context is either invoked or overlooked in storytelling, serving as a resource for conveying meaning. In turn, it becomes a shared reference point for social scientists seeking to understand actions and connect cases that might otherwise appear too disparate or disconnected.

This chapter is structured around two key questions. First, how diverse can the storytelling of intimate partner femicide be? In other words, to what extent can these stories depart from the dominant 'scripts'? This inquiry seeks to explore the degree to which these narratives

M. H. Di Marco, *Narratives of Femicide Perpetrators in Latin America*,
https://doi.org/10.1007/978-3-031-97367-3_7

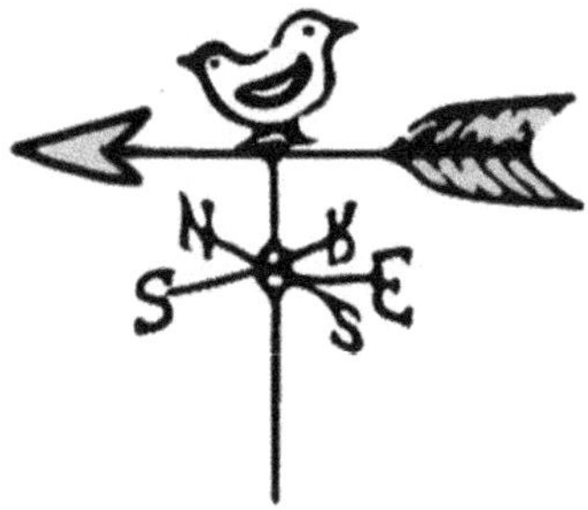

Fig. 7.1 Weather vane

can diverge from conventional patterns, and whether their components can still be traced back to broader narrative structures, even in cases that are readily psychologised or stripped of context. Second, how do these narratives incorporate—or fail to incorporate—context? This question is vital because these men come from different backgrounds and committed femicide at various points in time, influenced by distinct personal, social, and historical circumstances. Through this exploration, I aim to bring greater nuance to the analysis, highlighting the diversity of themes and narrative trajectories while critically engaging with the broader discussions introduced in earlier chapters.

The following vignettes highlight how social contexts are woven into the narratives of perpetrators, yet integrated in strikingly different ways. Alberto uses social context to depict a broad picture of rapid societal change, expressing a sense of being overwhelmed by "feminazis" and a perceived loss of personal agency. His narrative also underscores the influence of therapeutic discourses and the reconstruction of life stories from an institutional perspective. In contrast, Hugo completely erases the context. In his account, the femicide appears as an isolated, suspended event within their relationship, attributed solely to her actions and his blatant disregard for the lives of others. Finally, Aldemar offers what might be seen as a fragmented, disjointed narration of his life. While this narrative could be aligned with psychological labels such as schizophrenia, it nonetheless reveals contextual coordinates and deep-seated misogyny.

Alberto: Healthy Son of Patriarchy

I met Alberto through a social worker involved in the probation programme of a prison. For the past few years, Alberto had been attending a series of workshops focused on masculinities organised by a religious group closely associated with the liberation theology movement (Fig. 7.2). This was one of the few programmes I had encountered involving specifically intimate partner violence perpetrators. When we first met, he greeted me with a warm handshake, smiled, and engaged in casual chitchat. After I explained the research project and my interest in interviewing him, he responded with a nod and a smile, saying, "Well, of course. All talking is healing."

In his first interview, Alberto framed his life story as a downward spiral rooted in the abuse he endured as a child. Like other interviewees, his narrative served both as a means to rationalise the femicide and as an attempt to situate it within broader processes of personal and social victimisation—specifically, his experiences of childhood abuse and the pervasive influence of patriarchal structures:

> Like many people here [prison], I had a messed-up childhood. This isn't an excuse, but it's how I now understand things happened. It might not be enough for some people, like my family or children, but that's just how it is.

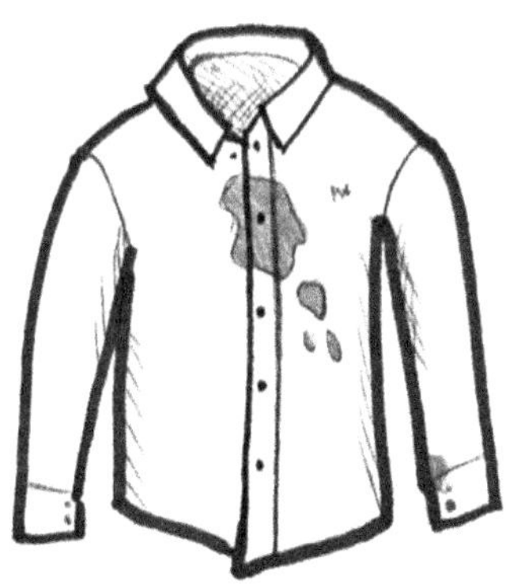

Fig. 7.2 Stained shirt

Alberto grew up in a middle-class household in the late 1970s. His father, a chemical engineer, was a regional manager for an international company, while his mother, previously an accountant, became a homemaker. As the eldest of three siblings, Alberto shared his painful experiences with his younger brother, Ramiro: "He was also a boy, so we had the same luck of being tortured." Their youngest sibling, a sister ten years younger, was spared much of their father's tyranny. "She was a girl and so young, so he let up. She was the little princess of the house."

His father's authoritarianism left deep scars, especially in his relationships with others. "It was a nightmare. I was paranoid about bringing someone over because it might set him off. But I was also anxious about being at a friend's house because he'd interrogate me about where I was and what 'bullshit' I was doing." Despite his father's oppressive behaviour, Alberto stressed that his childhood was not marked by a lack of material resources. He attended school, achieved good grades, and lived in relative stability.

In his teenage years, things eased slightly as his parents separated and his father moved to another city. This newfound freedom brought both relief and challenges. "At first, it was great, just a bit of hesitation, but great. Then I became very angry with some people, especially some female classmates. I thought it was just a normal phase, trying to get their attention, but things got rougher."

Alberto admitted to stalking and verbally abusing female classmates during this time. "There wasn't physical violence, but I was terrorising them, calling them names, hiding their stuff." This behaviour shifted when he met his first girlfriend. Initially full of romantic gestures, the relationship quickly soured as Alberto's jealousy consumed him:

> I was obsessed. Back then, people would justify chasing after your girl, and everyone supported it. So, I didn't think twice about following her, going through her things, even keeping a record of our sex life to spot changes. [...] It all ended when I got drunk, went to her house knowing her family wasn't there, caused a scene, and dragged her by the hair. The next week, it was over. Her brother came to beat me up. I felt ashamed, embarrassed, and guilty.

Right after high school, Alberto decided to get a tattoo of the Virgin Mary inked onto his thigh, calling it a gesture of reverence, particularly in intimate moments. He showed me the tattoo more than once, tying it to his faith and what he referred to as the "sacredness of women". Yet, when he spoke about it, I couldn't help but notice an underlying tension between his idealisation of femininity and a quietly pervasive misogyny. The tattoo, in essence, was a boundary—a way of marking respect, but also of situating women within a framework of purity and possession. For Alberto, this was not just any tattoo; it was the eternal symbol of the 'ideal' woman, one that belonged to him forever.

At university, Alberto began to distance himself from his father and made new friends while studying urbanism. However, his romantic relationships followed the same destructive pattern, marked by jealousy, stalking, and obsessive behaviour. When he met Ramona at a university party, the cycle repeated. "It was all over again. Different relationships, but the same pattern, right? I'd fall deeply in love, then get super jealous, then obsessed. The only difference was she didn't break up with me. So, we stayed together for years."

After moving in together, Alberto and Ramona started discussing having children. "I think, deep down, I thought: 'If she's pregnant and we become parents, she won't be able to leave me.'" They had two children, Dulce and Ramiro. Although Alberto did not describe himself as abusive towards them, he frequently referred to his short temper. "Having kids is a challenge, a very difficult one. It tests your patience, your temper, your ability to cope with sleep deprivation, and even your morals and values. Yet, it has changed me profoundly, for the better."

As the years passed, Alberto recounted how his life evolved alongside changing social contexts. Reflecting on the 2010s, he said: "I saw all those changes as a threat. I felt women were becoming aggressive. All that feminazi talk. Basic things, like giving a compliment or asking a girl out, were being demonised. It felt like society was crumbling, like this 'green wave,' as they call it, was taking over. I had an aversion to it."

A critical turning point came when Alberto's children became independent, and his wife began to redefine her social life after years devoted to family responsibilities. This transition unsettled their relationship, bringing insecurities to the surface. Alberto admitted to becoming increasingly controlling and aggressive as he struggled to adapt to the changes in their household. Over time, his frustrations escalated into episodes of physical violence, which he justified as stemming from his feelings of helplessness and the erosion of traditional family structures.

Ramona filed a complaint at the local police station following an incident that had deeply frightened her: he had threatened her with a kitchen knife. However, this did not escalate into a formal court case and remained at the level of a 'warning' issued by the police. "With one of those complaints, you end up 'marked' (*manchado*). It causes trouble because afterwards no one will hire you—it leaves you with a criminal record. That's for serious cases."

Alberto, in an attempt to avoid legal 'complications', voluntarily joined a batterer intervention programme. Several other interviewees also mentioned, in their own way, trying to outmanoeuvre a potential legal case for domestic abuse by attending these programmes. "At the time, I thought it was just a clever trick," he admitted. "I thought I could avoid legal trouble by appearing predisposed and well-intentioned. Obviously, it wasn't a good idea." Alberto attended two sessions before abandoning the programme altogether.

The femicide marked the tragic culmination of escalating violence. Frustration turned into physical abuse, anger became a means of instilling fear, and each cycle of violence repeated itself with guilt and renewed aggression. During a particularly tense conversation, Alberto's wife expressed a desire to take some time apart, which he interpreted as a definitive end to their relationship:

> And I lost it. I really, really lost it. One thing to make clear about how I was, I not only blacked out after that fight started. I remember going blind. Not blind-blind, but everything turned grey. I couldn't tell the difference in depth: walls, tables, everything seemed 2D, just shapes. I've talked about this as blinding patriarchy.

Alberto was reluctant to delve into the details of the day of the femicide, emphasising that revisiting it felt both painful and counterproductive. "It can have a harmful effect to go back to that day," he explained. Instead, he eagerly discussed his involvement in a masculinities programme, which helped him connect his experiences of victimisation with the abuse he perpetrated. "Sometimes I feel like a weather vane, driven by other forces—first my father's abuse, then patriarchy as a whole", he reflected.

* * *

From the outset of his narration, Alberto crafted a storyline that emphasised an 'etiology' of violence, framing his life as deeply marked by the interplay of personal history and patriarchal structures. His narrative centres on the profound impact violence has had on him, weaving together emotionally charged recollections of an abusive childhood and vivid accounts of abuse in his intimate relationships. He portrays himself as a man profoundly shaped by his circumstances, highlighting his lack of agency through the metaphor of a "weather vane", which he uses to describe the passive course of his life, swayed by external forces.

Alberto's use of this explanatory framework is notable for how it differs from other narratives collected in similar contexts. While some interviewees adopt narratives that focus on deflecting responsibility through victim-blaming or minimising their actions, Alberto's account leans heavily on institutional discourses to explain the roots of his violence. By invoking concepts such as childhood trauma and patriarchal norms, he situates his actions within a broader context of systemic failure and cultural conditioning. This strategy not only reinforces his claim of being shaped by forces beyond his control but also aligns his story with contemporary narratives that emphasise structural and institutional accountability.

His narrative, however, is not simply an act of self-exculpation. By drawing on these discourses, Alberto seems to be seeking a language that both rationalises his actions and allows him to process his experiences. His invocation of patriarchal structures, for instance, serves a dual purpose: on the one hand, it is a way to explain how his understanding of masculinity and relationships was shaped; on the other, it provides a means of critiquing the same system that perpetuated his sense of entitlement and control. Similarly, his detailed accounts of childhood abuse function as both a form of self-victimisation and a way of legitimising the argument that violence has been a defining, inescapable thread throughout his life.

Alberto's narrative thus reveals a complex interplay between personal responsibility and structural causation. His reliance on institutional discourses to explain the violence he inflicted suggests a conscious attempt to reconcile his identity as both a perpetrator and a victim. Yet, it also raises questions about the limits of such explanations, particularly when they risk overshadowing the agency he did exert in specific moments. In this way, Alberto's life story offers a compelling example of how perpetrators navigate the tension between owning their actions and attributing them to larger social and historical forces.

Hugo: The Widower

- Hugo: Would you like to hear about the killing first, or should I start by telling you about my life?
- Martín: What would you like to start with?
- Hugo: My growing years are quite interesting!

Hugo was undoubtedly a captivating interviewee. He was charming, well-articulated, and a wordsmith (Fig. 7.3). He was in his late sixties when we met, having already spent seven years in prison and traversed

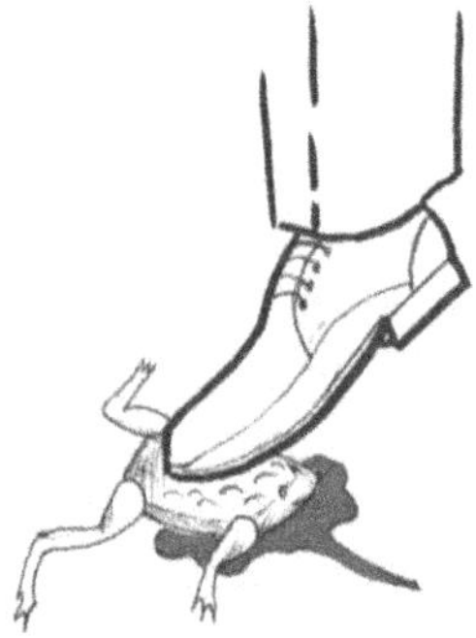

Fig. 7.3 Frog

several institutions along the way. Our initial conversation was memorable—not for what he said, but for how he said it. He was at ease discussing his life and felt content revisiting certain moments of his past:

> First and foremost, I am a physician. I have dedicated most of my life to treating patients, even here. Since there is a shortage of healthcare personnel in this unit, I help out whenever I can. After all, I'm in for the long haul! [Laughed].

Hugo was born in a sparsely populated province. His parents had relocated there from the capital in the 1940s due to the stable economic situation, as most jobs were tied to public administration. He described growing up in the province's second-largest city during the late 1950s as "incredibly boring".

> It was an incredibly boring childhood. There wasn't much to do. Even my sister and I, who'd never been anywhere else, knew that. Naps, walks, playing in the garden, and not even a tree to climb! [...] I just remember the dusty streets and the dry wind wearing them away bit by bit. The only interesting thing that ever happened was when the Jarjacha[1] got some poor one [girl] pregnant! That's why I didn't think twice about moving to the city as soon as I had the chance. [...] Looking back, it was the best decision I ever made – and the right one for the time, too. I ended up being the only one keeping things afloat, with the cheques I sent my father after he retired, and the money I spent at the pulpería when I visited.

At 17, he moved to the capital to study medicine. He lived in a small boarding house during his first years, still financially supported by his father. He described moving to the city as akin to discovering a new world, learning the ways of the people, transport, police officers, and locals. At one point, he even referred to himself as a peasant: "I was just learning the ropes, a humble nobody from the countryside, without a

[1] The jarjacha is a mythical creature from Andean folklore, often described as a hybrid of a human and a llama, created as divine punishment for committing incest or other grave immoral acts. Known for its terrifying "jar-jar" cry, it is said to wander at night, haunting isolated places and instilling fear as a cautionary figure in local communities.

penny to my name." However, his account of the following three years takes on a different tone, reversing this logic:

> I knew I had to meet people, the right people. So, in my first year of med school, I didn't lift my arse from the chair. I only studied. Once I got in, that's when the fun started, I joined the student union. And you can imagine a student union for medicine in the 1970s, it couldn't have been more political. But it was full of city boys, thinking they were clever, when all they could see was their own belly buttons. I had street smarts. I had travelled hundreds of kilometres to get there.

There are various ways people link events, creating a sense of progression. In Hugo's case, the arc was ominously majestic: he conquered cities, courses, and people. After joining the union, he swiftly rose through the ranks, becoming the right-hand man to the president. He viewed this as an opportunity to amass power and feel secure about potential jobs within the state. "This was a historic time of conquest, of gaining power for students, intellectual enrichment, and public health. I was there to gain momentum as well. We wanted a stronger state, but I wanted a role in it. Otherwise…", he smirked.

A few years later, Hugo completed his medical degree and specialisation. By then, he had already ascended the ranks as a lecturer at the faculty of medicine and secured a seat on the city's medical union board, a body that overlapped significantly with the faculty board members. Essentially, Hugo portrayed himself as a swift climber—an ambitious politician and a skilled physician.

During these years, he gave no indication of a stable intimate relationship. He spoke of brief flings and women he "had fun with", but they were described more as transactional, meeting a need at a particular moment. He briefly dated a fellow student, the daughter of a renowned professor, and had several encounters with women working in the union's administration before officially joining the board. It was not until he graduated and gained financial stability that he met Sandra. They were introduced through her father, an influential figure in the local government. At the time, Hugo was 27, and Sandra was just 18:

> You can tell a lot about a person by their parents. Sandra, for instance, was raised by a sharp, shrewd politician whom I admired greatly. He was highly educated, yet always operated in the shadows, a man with an imposing presence. Looking back, it seemed almost inevitable that she would end up with someone like me, someone, in many ways, not unlike her father.

Hugo's descriptions of people often hinged on whether he deemed them "smart" or "stupid", "resourceful" or "useless". In his view, Sandra was essentially a gateway to her father—valuable by association and, as he put it, "malleable." He saw her less as an individual and more as a tool he could shape to serve his ambitions:

> I took her out, and we started talking about politics. She sided with the workers, like me, but she didn't fully understand it. To her, it was just about rights and mobilising people. She couldn't see the bigger picture, it was about power, about building influence, about gaining momentum. That's when I encouraged her to join us in the union.

The following years were a whirlwind of events and travel—conferences, mobilisations, and institutional agreements. Sandra not only began working in the union but working *for* Hugo within it. This created a seamless overlap between their personal and professional lives, where work and home became indistinguishable.

After dating and cohabiting for four years, they married. She was 22; he was 31. Hugo showed me an old wedding photo, scanned and saved on his mobile phone (an item prohibited in prisons but nonetheless widely circulated in Latin American prisons). With a touch of irony, he remarked, "That was the start of my 'settled life.' A couple on paper, but a team in practice. She was indispensable, or rather, she made herself so."

He described their early years with a sense of nostalgia, though his version of "fond memories" seemed cold, devoid of any affection. Their home was a gathering point for political meetings, with Sandra playing the role of a gracious hostess, a partner in his ambitions. "She would entertain guests, handle the logistics, and smooth over the finer details," he said, casually noting, "I suppose she thought it was a sign of love. To me, it was just part of the setup."

Over time, Hugo's descriptions of their relationship hinted at an increasingly transactional nature. "She adapted well," he said with a smirk, as if amused by her transformation. "Sandra had her ideals, her principles, but I had a vision. I didn't have the luxury of idealism. She eventually understood that." His words reflected a man who viewed relationships as a means to an end, with people becoming malleable tools in his personal ascent.

They had two children in the early years of their marriage. He mentioned their births as milestones in a broader narrative, describing them as "additions to the family" without lingering on any emotional nuance. His story maintained the same self-centred tone, with the children's arrival fitting neatly into the timeline of his ambitions, as though they were inevitable extensions of his life's plan rather than transformative moments. There was no warmth or personal reflection; instead, he framed fatherhood as another role he took on with efficiency, a duty rather than a devotion.

In the hours of conversation that followed, Hugo recounted his rapid ascent with striking detail. He described moving from a modest medical practice and a position on the union's board to eventually heading the union for six years. His practice grew into a clinic, with him managing over a hundred employees. Yet his wife remained a mere supporting character in his story—a shadow on the periphery. I was struck by how little time he devoted to talking about his wife. Most men, even in distant retellings, tend to place their partners somewhere near the heart of the narrative. For Hugo, however, he alone was at the centre—a one-man solar system where everyone else orbited at a distance.

During one of our encounters, Hugo received a call—he had a visitor. He stepped out and returned twenty minutes later, casually referring to her as his "frog" (*rana*), a term used in some prisons to describe a prisoner's girlfriend, often carrying a derogatory connotation of promiscuity or filth. Hugo dismissed the situation with a nonchalant comment: "She can wait. I don't need anything today anyway." Then, as if reflecting on something deeper, he added:

> This is the problem with people. They don't understand how to navigate the world. They just think others will give them something or care for

them. No! One has to move like a fish in a school, get into the best current, and in that way, you gain actual power.

During our conversation, we also discussed a film we had both watched in the prison's improvised film theatre: *Luckiest Girl Alive*. In brief, the film follows a successful woman, soon to be married to her wealthy fiancé, who is forced to confront the trauma of an unpunished rape she suffered as a teenager when a documentary about a school shooting resurfaces her painful past.

> She was brimming with resentment, so full of spite! How many years had passed? Fifteen! Such a long time. Why return to it now, seeking revenge? I don't view her as a victim, no. I believe that incidents from the past, especially those that occurred during adolescence, should be understood within that context. What can she achieve now? Will putting him in prison erase it from history? Will it make her feel any better? No. I think she's motivated by spite and a desire for vengeance. "Why so much resentment for what he had done? He was a teenager. She is spiteful!" Love, on the other hand, is passion. "Passion is not quiet."

By our last session, Hugo had barely touched on the femicide itself. After recounting their marriage and raising the children, Sandra seemed to fade into the background of his narrative. Thirty years had passed between their marriage and the events he described with more detail, leading up to the femicide. Throughout his account, he did not describe any specific conflicts, arguments, or acts of aggression. Instead, there was a constant, underlying theme of control over the household and Sandra's daily life. The one issue that he repeatedly emphasised was her rebellious nature: "She always needed guidance; if not… she would just lose focus of things!".

During this last talk, however, he remarked:

> Everything is about perspectives. Some might see me as cold or calculating, but they're just kidding themselves, not knowing how to move in the world. Some might say I'm a killer, but if you think about it, I'm also a widower.

* * *

Hugo's life story could be the epitome of an ideal interviewee: almost a textbook case, replicating perfectly what academic papers and horror films alike often depict about killers. What sets Hugo apart is his blunt, unapologetic assertion that he feels no guilt for committing a femicide. Throughout our conversations, control—often expressed in a sardonic tone—was a recurring theme in his storytelling. Similarly, succeeding and positioning himself in powerful roles with social recognition were key drivers in Hugo's narrative.

Social change, evolving views on family and gender, are mentioned merely as background context, without any subjective implications for him. Even his direct and cold language regarding violence, coercive control, and the homicide itself presents a challenge to understanding, particularly in today's world, where language is far more surveilled, and political correctness has shifted the moral boundaries of speech.

Despite our eagerness to apply psychological labels, most of the narrative traits identified in the other stories are present in Hugo's account—albeit with a twist. Control over Sandra is central to the narrative but is framed as an instrumental aid to his life plan rather than a response to a fragile sense of self. Similarly, the breaking of gender norms is mentioned, but it is presented as being in service of 'something bigger' than Hugo himself. The weight of expectations, in his own way, lies at the core of the crime.

Hugo's account also brings to the fore the importance of age in shaping narrative transformation. While his bluntness is unusual—at least of this type—among the participants, older men in the group tended to use harsher, more visceral language and ideas, a topic that is later developed in depth (see this chapter). In this respect, Hugo resembles his peers more than the younger men. This underscores the need to recognise how time and age influence the construction of a life story, adding layers of meaning and shifting interpretations over time.

Overall, this narrative forces us into a paradox that challenges 'outlier' cases from a social sciences perspective, while simultaneously resisting the medicalisation of the interviewee. This raises the critical question: how can we—or should we—cross the boundaries between sociology and psychiatry? How do we understand the narrativisation such a complex case? Hugo's story challenges linear and universal interpretations of femicides, which are often viewed as unicausal and deterministic crimes. His story loops into itself, creating a closed narrative that traps us in a circular logic.

Aldemar: A Disorganised Story

Stories typically have a beginning, a climax, and a resolution, with protagonists and a recurring cast of characters (Fig. 7.4). When recounting an experience, we usually aim to convey meaning or create an impact on our listeners. As Bruner (1990) stated in *Acts of Meaning*: "They are a way of saying what a culture deems worth telling, and the form they take is that of the narrative practices of that culture" (p. X). However, Aldemar's story challenged this view.

Aldemar was the last man I interviewed for the project. At 59 years old, he had spent the past six years in a maximum-security prison, sharing a cell with just one other person—an unusual arrangement in the typically overcrowded conditions of Latin American prisons. According to his cellmate, all previous attempts to house Aldemar with others had failed miserably because few people could tolerate his "ways".

Aldemar's manner of speaking was circular: he would begin with a topic, expand, and branch out, then circle back to the initial theme.

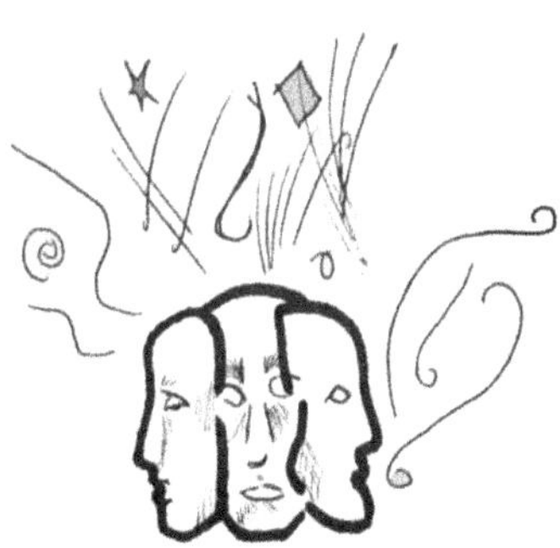

Fig. 7.4 Disorganised

These starting points were often grievances—an argument with a woman he once liked, a conflict with his father, or perceived unfair treatment by a prison officer. This peculiar narrative style, moving in loops, made it difficult to establish a clear order of events or discern what he deemed most significant.

In our first encounter, I explained the purpose of the project and the aim of the interviews, then asked him to share his life story—a standard opening for most of the interviews I had conducted. Typically, participants would frame their narratives around key life stages, often beginning with childhood or significant events such as the femicide. Aldemar, however, began with a quarrel involving a former girlfriend:

> I once had a girlfriend, Rita, who was very good. She was a very good person, a very good girlfriend. But she was too tempted by work. She would work extra hours, take new courses, always tempted to do more than was necessary. That's why I stopped it [the relationship]. She just didn't get it. Things have their place, you know? But she was always trying to change things, to make them different. That's not how it works.

Aldemar paused, focusing on fixing a cup of tea, before transitioning abruptly to a different topic: his father's character. The connection between his conflict with Rita and his reflections on his father remained unclear to me:

> You know, my father was a complicated man. He died years ago, but he was very smart and righteous. He always had a way of making things seem simple, even when they weren't. Since I'm not so smart, it always took me a while to get what he was saying. He would look at me, sometimes shaking his head, and say, 'Aldemar, you have to outsmart them. But you have to play by the rules.' He believed in rules, even when they didn't seem to work for everyone.

The first interview unfolded without a discernible structure. Aldemar spoke of his father, childhood memories, and even recounted his grandmother's funeral, which he claimed was mistakenly conducted in a Jewish cemetery instead of a Catholic one. His narrative drifted in unexpected directions, and many of the themes that typically emerged in these interviews across Latin America were conspicuously absent: there were no tales of harsh economies, no mention of gangs or friendships, no vivid descriptions of neighbourhood life. Instead, his account seemed detached from the social fabric that often anchors these stories, as if his experiences existed in a separate, insular reality.

In fact, most of these difficulty-related topics were more about portraying this reality—people and institutions—as nuisances or threats. His father's aggressive temper, the neighbours who failed to respect the boundary of the hedge, employers who disregarded limits, and overbearing friends all featured prominently. If there was a recurrent, albeit implicit, theme, it was avoidance and the pain associated with others.

In the second encounter, I reminded him of the purpose of the interviews. He nodded, but without altering his demeanour, responded, "I've always been a patient person. That's me. It's because of the Lord who has guided me. So when you talk to me, it's more like talking to Him. I'm here, but He…". He left the sentence unfinished, nodded slightly, and returned to his earlier story about Rita, adding a previously unmentioned detail:

> You know, Rita wanted me to change. She told me I had to be more... straightforward. But how could I? Things aren't straightforward. Life isn't straightforward. It's all tangled, like threads in a tapestry we can't see. God doesn't lay things out in straight lines; He works in patterns we're not meant to understand. That's why I told her. It's not me who's complicated, it's the world He made.

Aldemar's narratives were tangled too. They lacked the coherence typical of life stories, challenging the idea that people intuitively organise their accounts into linear, culturally recognisable forms. Instead, his stories were fragments—shards of memory and belief that resisted assembly into a cohesive whole.

In the third interview, Aldemar mentioned his wife, Julieta, for the first time. She was 16 years older than him, a fact he relayed casually, as though it were an unremarkable detail. They had met in the church choir; she was a widow at that point, having lost her husband several years earlier. Aldemar had not been married before. He spoke of their first meeting with a detached warmth, as if recalling a simple memory rather than the foundation of his later life. "We sang together every Sunday," he said. "It was just singing, nothing more. But there was something about her presence, something comforting."

Despite the significant age difference, their shared involvement in the choir created a bond that felt natural to him. Julieta's experience and wisdom contrasted with his own, as he described. "She didn't mind my quirks", Aldemar noted. "She understood the way I see things, even when I couldn't explain it myself." This initial connection in the choir laid the groundwork for their relationship, one that Aldemar approached with a sense of inevitability rather than conscious choice:

> She liked the way I saw things. She said I had a way of making her see what was underneath, you know? Like how a bird sees the ground from up high. She liked that. She said it made her feel closer to God, as if she could understand things she never thought about before. But I think she liked it too much, more than she should have.

His tone was neutral, as though Julieta were just another figure in his sprawling narrative. He spoke of her gardening, her strict routines, and her unexpected, childlike laugh. "She could laugh like a kid", he said.

Then, almost offhandedly, he mentioned her death. "It was too much," Aldemar said, staring at his hands. "I tried to explain it to her, but she didn't get it. And that was the end of it." He shifted slightly in his chair, his voice dropping to a murmur. "Some things can't be explained. Some things just happen, like a storm." When I asked him to elaborate, to fill in the large gaps in his account, Aldemar shifted to discussing a recent argument with a prison guard.

The lack of narrative resolution was unsettling. In most interviews, participants framed their actions—even violent ones—within moral, emotional, or situational contexts. They constructed explanations or justifications that fit broader cultural scripts about anger, love, or despair. Aldemar did none of this. His stories were not bridges to understanding but mazes with no clear exit.

By the last interview, it became evident that Julieta was both central to and absent from Aldemar's story. He spoke of her in fragments (moments of tenderness, flashes of frustration), but never as a whole person or shared life:

> She thought she knew what was best for me. But how could she? Nobody knows what's best for someone else. Not really. She kept pushing, telling me what I needed, but it wasn't her to decide. It was too much. Only God knows, right? Only He understands the path I should take, not her, not anyone else.

When I asked him what he meant by "too much", he gave me an unreadable look, his expression a mix of evasion and something I couldn't quite place. "Just too much", he said finally, as if those words were enough explanation. Then he added, "When I pushed her down the stairs, it wasn't just violence, it was an act of pushing her away from me." I could not help but interpret the act of pushing her down the stairs as a direct metaphor for how he had to distance himself from her and her radical ideas.

> Perhaps it is all about this movement of women. They forced her to push me, to pressure me, forgetting her place as a companion. She was supposed to be there for me, not take orders from other women. Only God can truly communicate an order, not these women and their ideas. Those movements, they forced her to think like them, to act like them. She wasn't supposed to be like that, not my woman. She was supposed to stand by me, not against me.

In the end, Aldemar's story resisted coherence, leaving me with more questions than answers. It was a narrative without a moral, a pastiche of moments that hinted at meaning without ever fully revealing it.

* * *

Ernest Hemingway famously wrote, "How did you go bankrupt? Two ways. Gradually, then suddenly" (2006 [1926], p. 126). In much the same way that Hemingway highlights the complexity of seemingly opposite alternatives coexisting, Aldemar's story brings to the forefront certain paradoxes of storytelling. On one hand, it pushes the boundaries of coherence, reminding us of the need to resist the inertia of Cartesian interpretations of narratives—stories are not inherently logical. People can be in a relationship and single at the same time, or both violent and peaceful within the same story. This is reflected in the disorganised nature of his storytelling, with fragmented patterns and unexpected verbal devices.

Even in this disorganised speech (which could be framed either as schizophrenic or simply as associative thinking packed with creativity), traces of dominant male-chauvinistic discourses emerge. Much like a chaos narrative (Frank, 1995), where the storyteller's suffering is so overwhelming that it resists narrative order and a sense of progress, it becomes difficult for both the teller and the listener to endure. Nevertheless, the morality expressed in the moments of lucidity regarding misogyny and threat remains "stable", despite the surrounding chaos.

On the other hand, Aldemar's narrative establishes an almost mechanical relationship between his crime and broader social change. He links his actions to the feminist movement, asserting that it was the root cause of his behaviour. He argues that "feminazis" have distorted fundamental moral values in society, deeply influencing his expectations of his family, his partner, and himself as a man. While his account differs in tone from other cases, it similarly highlights the tension between personal responsibility and social forces.

A third issue that emerged after conducting the interviews concerns the question of veracity. Some time later, I discovered that Aldemar had strangled his wife rather than pushed her, as he had originally claimed. Additionally, they had known each other for decades before their time in the choir; she had been a friend of Aldemar's mother. This raises a key question: how should we handle issues of truthfulness? To what extent can personal narratives, particularly those generated in institutional or carceral contexts, be trusted?

The value of oral testimonies, regardless of the field, does not rest solely on the factual accuracy of their content (Fujii, 2010). Instead, it often lies in the stories themselves, the underlying meanings shaping the responses, or even in what remains unsaid. Even lies, as Sandberg (2010) argues, hold value as vessels of meaning. This information is crucial because it illuminates how the current social and political landscape influences what individuals are willing or able to share with a researcher. Failing to consider this context risks analysts misinterpreting ambiguities, overlooking critical details, drawing flawed conclusions, or exposing informants to retaliation for their participation. Therefore, attending to the broader context is essential for safeguarding informants and developing robust explanations and theories about violence and its aftermath.

The crucial question here is: should narratives conform to our hermeneutic models, or should we develop new frameworks to understand the disjointed, incongruous stories people tell? Despite the abnormal discursive patterns—which might tempt some to resort to psychiatric labels to explain his case—the underlying narrative structure reflects core elements commonly found in the stories of many perpetrators. There is a strong tendency towards victim-blaming and, in his own teleological manner, a righteous self-presentation. However, his account lacks any meaningful engagement with relationships to explain his life history. Instead, a servile or instrumental understanding of intimate partners emerges when one probes beneath the surface of his speech.

Whynacht (2019) provocatively asks, "What do we do with the dangerous few?" This question often serves as the focal point in discussions of violence. Yet, as she argues, the question becomes more impactful—both theoretically and empirically—when shifted to focus on the majority, and the connections that link outliers to the broader population.

Outliers and Norms

In different ways, the stories of Alberto, Hugo, and Aldemar either intertwine with or break away from the social context embedded within their narratives. Some accounts overtly reflect male chauvinism, a total denial of responsibility, or, conversely, an absence of guilt, distinguishing them from others. In contrast, certain narratives place the individual's experiences of victimisation at the forefront, demanding the listener's attention. Others remain challenging to interpret—not merely ambiguous (Sandberg et al., 2015)—but incoherent and fragmented.

Psychologising and pathologising abuse might initially appear to offer a straightforward analytical lens to make sense of these stories. Hugo could easily be classified as a sociopath, given his lack of remorse and instrumental view of those involved in his 'play'. Aldemar might be described as schizophrenic, with disorganised speech marked by derailments and loose associations. Alberto, on the other hand, might fit the victim-perpetrator archetype, deeply traumatised by his abusive father.

However, adopting this medicalised perspective risks both depoliticising femicide as a structural phenomenon and undermining the potential for bridging the social sciences with mental health, thereby stalling the development of a more comprehensive hermeneutic framework. This critique does not aim to position sociology and psychology as oppositional disciplines; on the contrary, they can and should be epistemologically bridged to complement one another. Yet, the dominance of psychological frameworks in understanding violence is evident in how quickly we adopt their vocabulary and logic to decode these narratives.

This is not to deny the significance of mental health issues among perpetrators or their links to acts of violence. Rather, it is a call to resist the growing tendency to reduce what is fundamentally a socially embedded issue—shaped by cultural norms and power dynamics—to an individualised pathology. Such reductionism risks committing a level fallacy, wherein data or explanations from one analytical level are inappropriately applied to another.

Despite the outliers and contrasting features of these cases, they offer deeper insights into the narratives that foster femicide. In these vignettes, the ways in which context was incorporated into the stories varied significantly, yet the underlying logic of the violence adhered to familiar patterns. Themes of entitlement, punishment, future expectations, perceived damage, and threat emerged in distinct forms across the narratives. Whether influenced by delirium, psychopathy, or early traumatisation, the logic of harm remained consistent.

We might boldly assert that the narratives studied here share a core set of elements, which adapt to the subjective experiences of the perpetrators. These narratives can serve as a script for those lacking remorse, guiding cruelty and abuse; they can provide structure to an otherwise disoriented perception of reality; and they remain discernible, even though the layers of institutional reconstruction that often obscure them.

These stories illustrate that narratives are not suspended in isolation but are only comprehensible through—and because of—discourse. This analytical effort ultimately underscores a point emphasised in decades of language theory: we cannot understand any action without considering the performative effect of language, and thus social meaning and signification.

Part III

Deciphering the Recipes

"The average man is not directly interested in politics, and when he reads he wants the current struggles of the world to be translated into a simple story about individuals" (Orwell, 1941, p. 247).

Each of the vignettes presented in the previous chapters highlights distinctive elements involved in each crime. Hugo's blunt and instrumental view of relationships, Alberto's attempt to construct a persona reflecting his own abuse and victimisation, and João's navigation of a physically close-knit neighbourhood that remained passive in the face of his battering are all uniquely revealing. José's strategic navigation of institutional settings and Matías' heavy reliance on his friends further deepen this complexity.

These stories can certainly be read as singularities, each shaped by unique positionalities, from life histories to local and national circumstances. However, when considered together, they also form a broader picture of the narratives intertwined with these femicides. A broad-stroke interpretation of these stories would highlight distinctive narrative elements that contribute to femicide in the region. The key questions that arise are: Are there shared elements that illuminate the phenomenon as a whole? And are there distinctive patterns that differentiate the men?

In this part of the book, I examine three aspects of these stories in a transversal manner across Latin America, aiming to highlight how the common narratives underpinning femicide transcend individual subjectivities. In Chapter 7, I explore the shared threads in the stories to construct a narrative landscape of femicides. Rather than erasing nuances, by temporarily setting aside individual differences and national idiosyncrasies, we can identify the common mechanisms driving the phenomenon.

In Chapter 9, I investigate how these narratives have evolved across different generations of men. This exploration presents femicide (or femicides, as a heterogeneous phenomenon) as a dynamic process, with shifting narratives reflecting broader societal changes over time.

Finally, in Chapter 10 I seek to provoke the reader by illustrating how these stories may not be as far removed from their own moral frameworks as they might assume. Drawing on a pseudo-experiment inspired by breaching experiments in ethnomethodology, I test how swapping the genders or altering the ending of these stories influences (or does not influence) people's moral evaluations of these scripts. In essence, these chapters construct a structural portrait of these narratives, incorporate time and social change into our reading of this phenomenon, and highlight the widespread nature of such stories.

8
A Narrative Landscape

The Trauco, a mythical being from Chiloé Island in southern Chile, is described as a small, unattractive man with irresistible sexual power (Fig. 8.1). Said to seduce or assault women who wander alone in the forest, he serves as a convenient explanation for pregnancies without identifiable fathers. Similarly, the Jarjacha, an Andean shape-shifter cursed for committing incest, transforms into a ghastly creature—part human, part llama—that roams rural areas at night. El Pombero, found in Paraguay and Argentina, and El Tunchi, from the Peruvian Amazon, follow similar logics, punishing those—particularly women—who disobey certain traditions.

These folkloric myths share symbolic similarities: they attribute harm and blame to supernatural 'others' and provide pre-made scripts to explain socially censored events. Such narratives perpetuate cycles of violence by normalising these occurrences within society (Barán Attias, 2020). Crucially, these myths obscure gender-based violence by diverting accountability away from societal structures and reinforcing norms that justify and conceal violence against women.

To many, this folklore may seem far-fetched or incompatible with 'Western' rationalities. Hugo's allusion to the Jarjacha further underscores

M. H. Di Marco, *Narratives of Femicide Perpetrators in Latin America*, https://doi.org/10.1007/978-3-031-97367-3_8

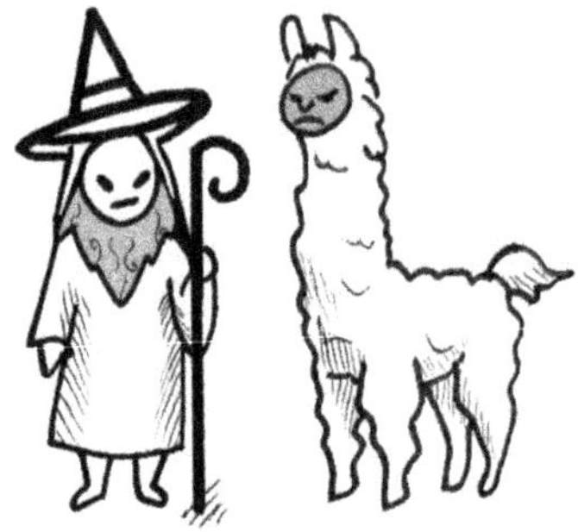

Fig. 8.1 Trauco and Jarjacha

the tendency to dismiss or belittle such myths (see Chapter 6.2). Yet, as anthropologists have emphasised for over a century, studying cultures different from our own can offer valuable insights into our own world-views. These myths, deeply rooted in specific cultural contexts, offer a vocabulary for articulating the unnameable. Similarly, the narratives of the men examined in this book function as explanatory scripts, shedding light on how they make sense of their actions and also the societal structures that shape them. If a language exists to legitimise killing a partner out of fear that she might leave, then such an act becomes conceivable. Just as the Trauco and Jarjacha share rationalising elements, so too do the stories told by these men. What, then, are the primary threats embedded in these narratives?

This chapter takes a broad approach to interpreting the men's stories, uncovering the 'recipes' that underpin their actions. I examine five key themes emerging from the vignettes—disruption, future and expectations, control, social support, and betraying narratives—highlighting a common pattern: their understandings of violence and gender are closely tied to rule-breaking and its punitive consequences. These narratives further reveal how expectations and assumptions about the 'future' play a crucial role in the dynamics of violence. Moreover, complicity, anticipated social impunity, and support from peers—as well as inactive or easily circumvented institutions—emerge as integral to the processes of sense-making and subsequent actions.

This analysis adopts a structural approach, deeply influenced by the concept of entitlement (Manne, 2020), to highlight shared themes—both latent and apparent—by focusing on the broader picture. Using methodological pointillism, where empirical observations serve as discrete yet interconnected data points, it prioritises common narratives over local nuances. While some subtleties are inevitably lost, this approach reveals the wider cultural and social dynamics embedded in these narratives.

A Shared Burden

Disruption

A structural theme in these narratives is the threefold concatenation of norm, deviation, and punishment. When men portray the characters in their stories, women are often positioned as being at fault—either for committing a direct offence against the perpetrator, their family, or the community. This goes beyond conventional victim-blaming, which typically focuses on the violence and coercive control itself (Ryan, 1971). Here, perceived rule-breaking is more comprehensive, encompassing a broader range of women's actions or omissions.

The centrality of norms should come as no surprise, as feminist scholarship has long established that misogyny is often a response to women's perceived violations of gendered regulations (Manne, 2020, p. 7). However, it would be a mistake to interpret this rule-breaking-and-punishment arc as an outlier narrative of 'monstrous men'. On the contrary, stories following this pattern appear to be widespread in anecdotes, memories, and popular culture—not only in the lives of these men but more broadly. These men are moralists (Segato, 2016), who see in their victims a moral deviation that demands sanction. Their actions, then, can be understood as attempts to enforce and reassert these norms.

Primarily, the narratives tied to rule-breaking adhere to a pattern of emotional pain transference, an argument we have made in the past (Fahs et al., 2023). Women's actions—such as seeking separation or autonomy, expressing divergent desires regarding parenthood, or asserting economic independence—or even their existence itself in some cases are interpreted by these men as acts of defiance or deviation. For most, these behaviours are framed as the root causes of their suffering, vulnerability, or emotional pain. Jorge, for instance, felt deprived of fatherhood following an abortion carried out without his consent; Celso portrays himself as wronged and a victim of immorality; similarly, Alberto describes feeling slandered when confronted with the possibility of a domestic violence complaint.

The failure to secure a perceived privilege or right is experienced by these men as a deep personal affront, reinforcing a sense of grievance. This mechanism lies at the heart of entitlement—the expectation that men have an inherent claim to certain social goods. Their narratives often unfold along a dual trajectory: the disruption of the status quo serves both as the dramatic climax of their story and as justification for casting themselves as victims. This framing is fuelled by feelings of despair, threat, and a perceived erosion of self. Most interviewees explicitly describe feeling belittled or persecuted by the legal system. The tension between their self-presentation as morally upright individuals and the legal system's insistence on their agency and responsibility compels them to actively resist institutional narratives, positioning themselves in opposition to legal and social accountability.

All of this can be understood as a power paradox: violence is enacted when power is perceived to be under threat (Presser, 2013). This framing challenges the assumption that violence arises from a position of stable power, instead highlighting how perceived instability can serve as the catalyst for its use. Perpetrators often perceive their violence as righteous—a means of transforming perceived harm into justice for "the people who used to be on top" (Cassino & Besen-Cassino, 2021, p. 10). It also sheds light on how something as vast and abstract as patriarchy is enacted in everyday, face-to-face interactions.

This understanding of violence compels us to consider *when* these narratives are enacted. While the interviews provide a post facto picture (both of the homicide and the imprisonment), thinking dynamically about the relationship between violence and power suggests that the relevance of the narrative becomes acute when change is perceived. Narratives—ever-present and adaptable—are employed situationally. As

Rose (2021) points out, violence serves as a stark reminder of the fraudulence of the perpetrator's power. Thus, violence becomes an instrumental tool in these stories for reclaiming what is perceived as rightfully theirs.

Alternatively, narratives about rule-breaking can be understood not merely as responses to perceived threats but as attempts to forge emotional connections. This perspective requires examining not only how these men reacted to instability in the status quo but also how they initially formed intimate relationships. Hugo and Matías, for example, vividly describe bonds in which control itself was the foundation of intimacy, with violence and abuse serving as mechanisms for creating a sense of emotional security and stability.

This reading of their stories challenges a predominantly restrictive understanding of violence, aligning with the canonical distinction between positive and negative dimensions of power (Foucault, 1990). Violence may not solely be a mechanism of repression but also a productive force—one that generates knowledge, norms, and identities. While much of social science has adhered to the first hypothesis—interpreting power relationally but largely as a reactive and oppressive force—this alternative view, in which aggression and control function as tools for shaping social bonds, offers an additional layer of insight often forgotten. Such a reading broadens our understanding of power dynamics in these narratives, highlighting how mechanisms of control are not merely reactive but can also be instrumental in shaping the contours of intimate relationships. This approach invites us to rethink how power operates within relational contexts, moving beyond simplistic dichotomies of oppression and resistance.

The men in these scenarios embark on an 'intimate salvage' mission, drawing on whatever resources are available to them—reinforced by enabling narratives—to restore what they perceive as a disrupted order. By labelling their partners as wrongdoers or victimisers, they invert the situation, positioning themselves as the true victims. In this process, misrecognition (Wacquant, 1989) plays a crucial role, as power dynamics are reframed in ways that obscure their actual nature. Recognising violence as such—previously normalised—demands a deliberate and often difficult effort.

In these vignettes, violence emerges not merely as a reactive or impulsive act but as an instrument embedded in the relational and situational contexts of these men. As an instrumental action, aggression becomes a means of addressing disruptions in perceived order, whether intentional or accidental. Lethal violence, in particular, functions as an act of 'repair', restoring a sense of self that has been destabilised. This restoration extends beyond the individual to include others—friends, neighbours, or a broader social circle—highlighting the collective dimension of these narratives. Ultimately, the validation of one's identity through others' perceptions, what Cooley (2010 [1902]) termed the 'looking-glass self,' is central to understanding both the scope and justification of violence in these accounts.

For these men, violence was not only a tangible, physical act but also a narratively legitimate one—a means of making sense of their experiences and actions. Their accounts often framed violence as the only available option, camouflaging the lack of perceived alternatives. This framing carried an aura of immediacy and inevitability, portraying violent responses as bodily reactions rather than deliberate decisions. Such narratives underscore the importance of interrogating the interplay between a perceived inevitability and the deliberate construction of justification within their stories.

Future

The flipside to rule-breaking in these narratives is time. In many forms of harm, the expectation that an action, whether deemed justifiable or not, will produce specific outcomes is a key component. Temporality, therefore, reveals how these actions are anchored in past experiences, shaped by present goals and values, and directed towards anticipated events. Much like vicarious violence—a form of harm in which one person harms another by targeting a third party, often a loved one, to exert control or inflict psychological suffering (Bancroft et al., 2011)—femicides are carried out with the expectation of reshaping relational dynamics.

It should be apparent that a central aspect of temporal structuring in these narratives is the projection of the future. Femicide often emerges as a response to an event that disrupts an anticipated life trajectory—an interruption of the imagined future (Enander et al., 2021). It can be seen as a funnel, where expectations, emotions, and actions converge towards a single, inescapable event. Whether it involves a divorce, the revelation of an affair, a wife leaving for work, or even something seemingly trivial, like a cake, these occurrences mark ruptures in the anticipated future. By their nature, they create irreconcilable contradictions between what the perpetrator and victim desire, fundamentally altering the project of the relationship (Dobash & Dobash, 2015) and destabilising the men's vision of the future.

For these stories to have an effect, they need to be reinforced by the absence of narrative alternatives. When expectations centre on a specific moment—such as Matías feeling let down and abandoned, Celso feeling betrayed, or José discussing custody and harbouring resentment for being left—participants rarely mention viable options to circumvent aggression. More commonly, emotions, expectations, and tensions are compressed into a singular, pivotal moment. This narrowing of possibilities does not merely reflect actual options but underscores the emotional styles of familicidal perpetrators (Websdale, 2009), who often struggle to process emotions such as shame, rage, fear, and anxiety. In their eyes, there are few, if any, alternative ways to confront their conflicts.

Overall, these men interpreted certain moments in their intimate relationships as negative turning points. More notably, for them, disagreement and splitting up are synecdoche for humiliation and despair, much like 'Band-Aid' is for a bandage. This points to the narratives available to them to interpret these 'disagreements' as such, showing the symbolic repertoire they have to make sense of their lives.

The absence of thinkable, narratable, or emotionally viable alternatives is a defining feature of femicide narratives. It reveals how the perceived inevitability of events—shaped by rigid expectations and a lack of conceivable resolutions—directs the story's trajectory. The 'knots' of these narratives, where everything culminates, leave no space for alternative outcomes, reinforcing the tragic inevitability embedded in their structure. This interplay between the narrative climax and the absence of alternatives highlights how storytelling frames the perceived options and emotional pathways available to the characters.

Despite these disruptions and crushed expectations, perpetrators often describe experiencing a sense of closeness to the victim while simultaneously mourning the loss of their shared 'life projects'. This duality underscores the connection between temporality and violence, revealing how narratives of harm are deeply entwined with the construction and deconstruction of imagined futures.

Control

In *Milkman*, Anna Burns (2018) instrumentalises the notion of encroachment to evoke a quiet yet relentless violation of the protagonist's personal space, where a man's presence (the milkman) seeps into her life like an uninvited shadow. This slow, almost imperceptible invasion instils a palpable sense of terror, as the protagonist struggles to define the nature of the intrusion. Yet, it steadily undermines her autonomy, reflecting the insidious nature of power that operates through both silence and subtlety:

> At the time, age eighteen, having been brought up in a hair-trigger society where the ground rules were—if no physically violent touch was being laid upon you, and no outright verbal insults were being levelled at you, and no taunting looks in the vicinity either, then nothing was happening, so how could you be under attack from something that wasn't there? At eighteen I had no proper understanding of the ways that constituted encroachment. I had a feeling for them, an intuition, a sense of repugnance for some situations and some people, but I did not know intuition and repugnance counted, did not know I had a right not to like, not to have to put up with, anybody and everybody coming near. (Burns, 2018, p. 6)

Similarly, in the stories of perpetrators, control emerges as a central theme, functioning as the counterpart to punishing deviation. Dominance and oversight become necessary for surveillance and planning future actions. However, its meaning varies across the different narratives told. Control may involve monitoring, identifying, and addressing a perceived threat, encompassing pre-emptive aggression, or even being framed as a form of pedagogical action. For some men, the idea of control is inseparable from those of love or romance. These shapeshifting meanings of control define the contours of the stories, highlighting how narratives create tailored scripts that interact with local cultures and institutions on a deeply intimate scale.

Perpetrators often frame their actions as expressions of entitlement, responsibility, or protection, aligning with traditional masculine ideals that objectify women and restrict their autonomy. In this context, control is presented as a relational performance, where actions such as isolation or surveillance respond to perceived threats to authority, shaped by societal expectations and personal insecurities. Tactics like social confinement not only maintain control but also silence the victim, reinforcing a cultural narrative that diminishes women's agency and justifies violence, with femicide emerging as the ultimate act of silencing.

These narratives of control typically follow five main structures. *Fear of loss or betrayal* often justifies pre-emptive control, driven by insecurities such as fears of infidelity or abandonment, with blame projected onto the partner for failing to reassure or for challenging male authority. *Externalisation of responsibility* occurs when control is attributed to social or cultural factors, such as upbringing or societal expectations (e.g., "That's how I was raised"), or external pressures like stress or substance abuse, allowing men to deflect personal accountability. *Silencing the victim* involves invalidating the partner's concerns, framing objections as overreactions, and controlling the narrative to reinforce isolation and suppress dissent. In this arc, silencing—from Héctor's forced medication to Alberto's body terrorism—becomes a tool for managing disruptions to their expectations. *Peer reinforcement* is evident when narratives include peer approval of controlling behaviours, reinforcing them as part of a shared understanding of masculinity. Finally, *shifts in accountability* may arise in therapeutic or intervention contexts, where men partially acknowledge their behaviour but avoid full responsibility. Some also cast themselves as victims, focusing on their own struggles rather than their actions.

These narratives primarily focus on explaining the control exerted. Nonetheless, these actions—i.e., manipulation, gaslighting, interference with social relationships, physical abuse—were often framed as something other than control. For these men, these were not stories of control but rather stories of obstacles, challenges, and strategies to overcome. On one hand, this may imply that most of these stories align with what Hearn (1998) famously placed on the spectrum between repudiations, excuses, and justifications. There is, in general, no concessions: no acknowledgement of wrongdoing. On the other hand, it may indicate that, within these social settings, control was not thematised explicitly as such.

The open challenge now lies in stating, point-blank, that for the men who committed this harm—and potentially for many others—control is understood through a different lens. It might be seen as emotional intensity, or as a less appreciable personality trait. It might even be seen as a sign of care and love. A second challenge emerges when we highlight that at least one type of narrative involved in performing abuse is inextricably linked with peers. Strategies designed to restrict freedom are not solely grounded in narratives about gender and women; they are equally tied to stories about networks.

Support

> A way of seeing is also a way of not seeing – a focus upon object A involves a neglect of object B. (Burke, 1969, p. 70)

In a similar vein to Burke's argument, our focus on certain mainstream types of femicide stories often excludes complementary ones. The heterogeneity of narratives told by perpetrators extends beyond intimate relationships or the victim herself, involving a broader set of characters, such as friends, relatives, neighbours, police officers, and bureaucrats. These networks play various roles in the narratives; at times, they are secondary actors, while at other times, they are pivotal in explaining turning points in the lives of perpetrators, even when unrelated to the femicide itself. For some men, however, peers hold a crucial position in the crime itself.

There has long been interest in understanding how social relationships shape violence. Some have approached this through the lens of social capital and networks, while others have focused on kinship and peer dynamics. Regardless of the terminology, theories centring on networks—most notably male peer support (DeKeseredy & Schwartz, 2013)—have a common focus on the connection between perpetrators' social circles and their misogynistic attitudes and practices. And yet, these perspectives are often overlooked when addressing intimate femicide.

From a narrative perspective, this calls for examining stories about peers—their support, complicity, and, to some extent, impunity. Examples abound in the vignettes presented in this book. Matías, for instance, recounted relying on his friends for validation and, in extreme situations, for evading detection. João's dismissal of feeling threatened by his neighbours' potential intervention was rooted in a sense and assumption of impunity, tied to the perceived sanctity of 'domestic problems'. Similarly, José's narratives about navigating bureaucratised institutions illustrate how social mechanisms helped him block potential early interventions. In Héctor's vignette, the psychiatrist friend who prescribed pills played a pivotal role in this dynamic. In contrast, in Jorge's story, the repair shop boss stands out for his inaction by failing to report the fighting until the very last occasion.

Examining the meta-data from the interviews—the laughter, omissions, and tones (Fujii, 2010)—can also illuminate the extent to which these stories of support are embedded in these narratives. Silences regarding the potential intervention of friends, the omission of names, and the romanticisation of male kinship and bonding form the backbone of many of these accounts. For example, Sergio's story uncovers an underlying eroticisation of his relationship with his cousin, coupled with blind trust in his cousin's support, which makes his actions more intelligible. The story of aggression becomes clearer when we recognise how Sergio's worldview—as conveyed through his narrative—is reinforced by a storyline that amplifies his confidence.

A productive lens for analysing these narratives is homosociality (Bird, 1996; Sedgwick, 1985). These men do not live in social isolation; their connections with others shape both their lives and their stories. Nor are their narratives uni-focal; they often rely on intertwined accounts involving peers and networks. Loyalty, pacts of silence, and looking the other way become operative elements in this dynamic. Male support networks, therefore, are crucial to understanding, on one hand, the stories that foster violence, and on the other, those that minimise the severity of intimate partner violence, promote victim-blaming, and ultimately justify 'helping' a friend.

Ultimately, the important role that others play in stories about femicide points to the undercurrent of a *narrative of complicity*, revealing different scenarios: 'My friends will stand by me to help me', 'People will judge me if I don't act', 'Institutions will not meddle in this private business'. This complicity can be seen as a crucial link in the chain of impunity, reflecting moral reasoning (Whynacht, 2019). It may, as mentioned above, form a vital part of social support mechanisms. More broadly, it may be understood as a necessary element in legitimising violence.

Even when characterised by denials, lies, errors, or omissions, these stories reveal much about the men's expectations and values. In this regard, Plummer (2019) theorises collaborative narratives, which expand our understanding of how these accounts are co-constructed through relationships and shared meanings. This raises an inevitably, yet counterfactual question: could intimate femicides have occurred without the presence of narratives of complicity? Are machista discourses focused solely on women sufficient to explain these acts of violence?

Betraying Narratives

Part of the argument developed in this book is that femicides can only occur if the narrative landscape permits them. This aligns with the broader theory of the effects of discourse: for an action to take place, or even be thinkable, discursive conditions must exist to provide the words, imagery, and (see Presser, 2013; Presser & Sandberg, 2015). Among the narratives I highlight, some point to and embody a sense of impunity and trust in existing complicities. This is a robust claim from a narrative standpoint, as it reflects a belief in a social practice rooted in stories.

I would, however, challenge orthodox approaches in narrative studies by making an epistemological leap between narratives (the telling of words) and practices (the behaviours described by those words). The interviews analysed here may not only reflect the legitimisation of violence against women and the web of complicities involved in this—stories that enable men to support each other, 'turn a blind eye' to violence, or engage in victim-blaming—but also can reveal the mechanisms at play within friendships and acquaintanceships, as well as within specific institutions, such as police stations. This could, for example, signal the logics underpinning himpathy, the tendency to empathise more with male perpetrators of harm than with victims (Manne, 2017). The epistemological leap, therefore, lies in bridging narrative understanding with a realist analysis of the practices these interviews expose.

Complicity narratives, in particular, provide a critical lens for examining the practices of individuals, especially male friends and peers. For instance, Matías' description of a cover-up and Héctor's reliance on a physician friend to secretly medicate his wife illustrate how trust, as conveyed in these stories, was deeply intertwined with the femicides they committed. These stories not only expose the actions of the perpetrators but also highlight the roles played by their friends. Complicity is, thus, not merely a narrative phenomenon but also a material one, manifesting itself in concrete practices.

The stories told by these men can be partially understood as by-products of social learning and face-to-face interactions. This situates the analysis of narratives within social settings and relationships. Scholarship on these social dynamics has shown how spaces of peer socialisation—pubs, sports teams, gangs, workplaces, and childhood friendships—can shape certain forms of intimate partner violence. In essence, narratives are shaped by informational support—the "help in defining, understanding, and coping with problematic events", also described as advice, appraisal support, and cognitive guidance (Cohen & Wills, 1985, p. 313). Whether peers' actions are seen as support or a response to abuse (Berggren & Gottzén, 2022), acknowledging their role helps to further decentre the discussion of femicide from the 'private' sphere.

Ultimately, this perspective requires bridging basic assumptions in narrative research and, more importantly, questioning the unidimensional aspect of femicide narratives. By connecting stories with the societal realities in which they are conceived and reshaped, we may better understand the interplay between storytelling and the social structures that enable violence.

Connecting the Stories: Narrative Tessellation

In *Why War?*, Philip Smith (2005) argues that every war has its roots in the way stories are told and interpreted. His understanding of belligerence challenges dominant perspectives that focus solely on the struggle for resources. Yet conflict and violence—on any scale—are inextricably tied to processes of sense-making. This argument extends further, emphasising that meaning does not exist as isolated signification but as part of a wider frame that connects these meanings into a coherent scheme. Put simply, it is not only the meanings attributed to femininity that might explain violence against women, but also the connections between femininity, masculinity, hierarchies, and desirability, for instance. These connections are embedded within stories.

Interestingly, a similar metaphor has been used to discuss violence against women. Segato (2016) famously described the killing of women in Latin America as a war against women. This metaphor is more useful than simply viewing gendered violence in a straightforward way. On one hand, war is seen as a strategy for controlling resources, a way of organising power. On the other, it reflects how patriarchal systems and masculine identities engage with difference—asserting control over what they cannot fully understand or dominate (Benjamin, 1988). Femicide may reveal how dominant rationalities fail to recognise women as fully human subjects. Violence against women, then, is not just about power but also about a fundamental failure to see women as equals. Psychoanalytically, this is not merely the problem of the 'other', but of the unattainable—the ungraspable, that which resists full control and comprehension.

This work assumes that the stories told by these men can be instrumentalised to understand social structures. The fact that similar stories are told across the region should shift our attention away from the individuality of specific cases and from a non-agentic understanding of patriarchy. Instead, it may refocus our analysis on how existing narratives shape femicide: men told their stories, each with its own nuances, drawing upon the narrative templates they had encountered before.

From a bird's-eye view, the repetition of these stories forms a *tessellation*: a network of interwoven narratives that fit together without gaps, creating a structured whole. However, a bottom-up approach would focus on how individual actions and the rules they enact (e.g., "I perceive her resistance as overwhelmingly aggressive, and physical violence is a legitimate response to counteract her") generate a pattern of repetition. The accumulated actions construct a broader structure, aligning with a more dynamic understanding of narratives. As Ahmed (2004) argues, stories do not merely reflect social phenomena; they actively shape them through their circulation, influencing how we feel and respond.

Understanding femicide as a product of such tessellations points to the interconnectedness with broader supporting narratives, rather than its singularity. When men discussed their crimes, they were not confined to solely talk about women; they spoke of their own lives, friendships, institutions, work, football, and politics. Recognising the interwoven nature of these narratives should encourage us to think more systematically about this narrative connective tissue. Discussions of masculinity are rarely separable from those of femininity; thresholds for harm doing and the discourses available on the instrumentality of violence are inextricably linked. To disentangle these elements risks reducing the phenomenon to an overly fragmented, cubist interpretation.

This argument contends that too much research isolates specific aspects of femicide. Acknowledging the tessellation could foster a more systemic understanding of their reproduction and interconnectedness. Integrating narratives of entitlement with stories that reinforce impunity, for instance, could be a vital step towards developing more realistic long-term prevention strategies. This perspective is particularly relevant in contemporary times, when extensive research has focused on specific facets of this phenomenon, and prevention strategies have largely been fragmented (e.g., UNODC & UN Women, 2024, p. 22). Rather than dissecting individual factors in isolation, this approach should bridge different elements to reveal a more comprehensive picture. Femicide is undoubtedly not only about women; it is also about the trust that violence against women will go unpunished, among other factors. Certainly, the actions of aggressors are entwined with the inaction of peers who fail to intervene.

Another question prompted by this lens: can we truly understand the killing of women solely through stories about women, without also considering narratives about the reliability of institutions? Counterfactual reflection could aid analytical thinking here. While theoretically flawed, such hypotheses help illustrate connections: what if João had feared being confronted by his neighbours? What if José had perceived the police as impartial and committed to due process? Without external support, would Hugo's covert medication of Priscila have been possible? Faced with these questions, what is omitted, taken for granted, or left unsaid by these men can provide crucial insights into their narratives. These omissions, for instance, challenge the notion of a rational, omniscient, and chameleonic storyteller. Conversely, they reveal that narrators are not entirely in control of what they disclose.

There exists, at its core, a catechism of stories that establishes scenes, characters, values, and plots with beginnings, middles, and ends. This seemingly dominant grammar of storytelling and metaphor creation—the medium through which we structure our worldview (Lakoff & Johnson, 1981)—is what sets the stage for femicides to become thinkable and actionable. Within these elements, disruptions of gender norms, expectations, control, support, and group dynamics emerge as foundational pillars for decoding the coda of such narratives. This, in turn, should draw our attention to both the problem of the stories told by men and the stories we construct to explain these heinous crimes. As Chimamanda Adichie (2009) beautifully elaborates, this is the *dangers of the single story*: "The single story creates stereotypes, and the problem with stereotypes is not that they are untrue, but that they are incomplete. They make one story become the only story" (p. 12).

9

Comparing Apples and Pears: The Issue of the Historical Moment

> Nobody is ever the same as anyone else who ever lived, lives, or will live. This uniqueness is revealed only in acting and speaking, and it is this revelation—this expression of oneself in deed and word—which makes one's own appearance in the human world. (Arendt, 2018 [1958], p. 8)

At its core, this chapter is shaped by two central questions: Do the stories of these Latin American men follow consistent patterns across generations? And what insights do the variations in their storytelling styles—what might be described as their 'narrative voice'—offer about our current historical moment in the context of femicide? Earlier sections of this book adopted a pointillist approach to identifying narrative patterns, using this strategy to provide a broad understanding of femicide and revealing what Plummer (2019, p. 43) describes as a "canopy of human values". However, such a strategy inevitably simplifies the complexity of the phenomenon—not all stories conform to the same patterns (Fig. 9.1). While this cross-cutting lens offers valuable insights, it also risks obscuring the differences between shifting accounts.

This issue is particularly salient when considering time—not only because the social sciences have often overlooked this dimension, but

M. H. Di Marco, *Narratives of Femicide Perpetrators in Latin America*,
https://doi.org/10.1007/978-3-031-97367-3_9

Fig. 9.1 Apples and pears

also because studies of violence risk producing overly static and bleak portrayals if they fail to incorporate change as a factor in the analysis. Interestingly, current discussions on femicide have largely focused on its identification and measurement, and its legal recognition and criminalisation. By contrast, there is a longstanding body of scholarship on intimate partner violence and change, which has placed social transformation and desistance at the heart of its discourse. This bifurcation into two distinct fields of literature raises a pressing question: do the narratives of femicide perpetrators remain consistent over time in Latin America?

Time, therefore, becomes the central focus of this chapter, which seeks to trace certain threads of change within these narratives. This chapter explores the shifting narratives of femicide through the lens of generational differences, examining both the ages of the men and the historical periods in which they lived before committing femicide. The analysis centres on men born in the 1950s–1960s, 1970s–1980s, and 1990s–early 2000s (n = 8, 20, and 27, respectively), with a focus on comparing their experiences within the historical context of their lives. The underlying premise in the analysis is straightforward: while the temporal context in which these stories are constructed may be similar, being born and raised in different eras—such as the 1960s compared to the early 2000s—inevitably shapes the narratives perpetrators produce. Their attempts to rationalise their actions draw on distinct discursive resources shaped by their respective social and historical contexts.

The chapter puts forward two main arguments. First, the ways in which younger and older men narrate their accounts of femicide differ significantly. Second, these evolving styles of storytelling offer insights into broader processes of change in perpetration in Latin America or, at the very least, in the cultural scripts that sustain it. These changes are likely shaped by a combination of institutional pressures, media portrayals, individual biographical trajectories, and local social dynamics. They also reflect transformations in the narratives that normalise femicide and its perceived legitimacy. Notably, these narratives appear to evolve in three distinct ways: a shift from reactive and self-righteous justifications to more apologetic accounts; a softening of the language used to describe acts of violence; and a diminishing reliance on discourses of implicit impunity, accompanied by an increasing support for punishment intertwined with justificatory narratives. By examining these changes, this chapter seeks to initiate a long-overdue discussion on how perpetrators and their stories evolve over time.

Apples: Older Stories, Firmer Tales

Celso and Hugo serve as telling examples for examining the intersections of narrative and historical context. These two vignettes are composites of men born in the late 1950s and early 1960s, placing them in their mid to late sixties at the time of the interviews. Raised in starkly contrasting social circumstances—Celso in a small, vulnerable rural town with limited access to basic rights, and Hugo in relative economic comfort with rapid social mobility—it is unsurprising that their life trajectories diverged sharply. Celso became a manual labourer with minimal social security and limited support, while Hugo pursued a career as a physician, often holding positions of high authority.

Despite these differences, their stories show striking similarities with those of other men from their generation. Celso described his partner's behaviour as "misbehaving", exhibiting a "bad attitude", and engaging in morally reprehensible actions. Hugo, on the other hand, characterised his partner as an obstacle to his ambitions. Like many men of their generations, both recounted their stories with directness and bravado. Their descriptions of violence, which ranged from extreme coercive control—such as covertly medicating their spouse—to severe manipulation and gaslighting, were heavily and self-righteously justified. This framing presented their aggression as a form of moral defence, where violence was rationalised as necessary to restore order.

Older perpetrators, such as Celso and Hugo, frequently rationalised their violence as a means of re-establishing discipline within the relationship, articulating their motivations in a notably direct and ostentatious manner. Celso, for example, unapologetically described his abuse: “She was constantly testing my limits, and I had to put a stop to it. If I didn’t, she would have walked all over me in every argument we had.” While such justifications may contain multiple layers, the stark bluntness of these statements is striking. Rule-breaking emerged as a recurring theme in all the stories, but the directness with which these men expressed it stands out as a defining characteristic of this cohort. This justification, rooted in a desire to reassert control, often appeared more calculated than the impulsivity typically associated with younger perpetrators. Whereas younger men may act out of a sense of ‘emotional urgency’, older men tended to frame their actions as deliberate measures to maintain the status quo within their relationships.

Interestingly, despite a degree of self-reflection, older perpetrators rarely framed their stories around remorse. This does not suggest an absence of remorse per se—an important aspect in other areas of study—but rather that their narratives did not emphasise this issue. Instead, they portrayed their violence as a justified response to their partner’s behaviour. Héctor, for example, rationalised his actions by stating, “She pushed me to the edge. I didn’t want to hurt her, but she wouldn’t listen. I had to do something.” His justification reflects a deep-seated belief in the necessity of maintaining dominance within the relationship. Like him, other men were less likely to question the legitimacy of their control over their partners, seeing it as an integral part of their masculinity and authority.

These men also tended to frame their actions in terms of *regret for the consequences* rather than the acts themselves. This was a central discursive movement in these stories: “I regret what happened, but I regret that it went too far. I just wanted to make her understand, to teach her a lesson.” This statement underscores a key distinction: while younger men often deny responsibility for their actions, men born in the 1950s and 1960s express regret for the outcomes, though they still justify the violence as a necessary corrective measure. For them, violence remained an acceptable tool for resolving conflicts and maintaining control, even as they acknowledged the harm caused.

Their narratives often described relationships as increasingly strained over time, with *power imbalances* becoming more pronounced. "We used to be fine, but over the years, she started to get too independent", one interviewee stated. Another added, "Her obsession with going back to work was ruining everything." The loss of control was often attributed to their partner's growing autonomy, leading them to justify their violence as a response to perceived defiance. Unlike younger men, who may view their partners as passive recipients of control, older men were more likely to see their partners as active agents challenging their authority.

However, their accounts also revealed a sense of *resignation or weariness*. Many described their violence as a last resort after years of attempting to maintain control through other means. "I tried everything to make her listen, but nothing worked", one man said. Another reflected, "What else could I have done at the time?" This resignation suggests that violence was not always their first option but rather a final, calculated effort to restore a sense of order in their relationships. The shift from calculated action to impulsivity reflects a different understanding of the overall aggression, where men born in the 1950s and 1960s feel an increasing urgency to preserve their authority.

A final notable feature of their narratives was the implicit sense of impunity. As I argued previously (see Chapter 6), stories of femicide perpetration not only reflect these men's actions but also the network of other actors involved in their everyday lives. Fear of detection—whether by relatives, institutions, or law enforcement—was rarely a theme in its own right. Instead, their stories conveyed a strong sense of entitlement to act aggressively. Strategies to avoid detection or to socially isolate their partners were not central themes. To some extent, this was a less pressing concern for them and, in parallel, an element taken for granted by the characters of their stories: abuse can go unnoticed. This backdrop of assumed impunity underscored their narratives, highlighting the normalisation of violence within their accounts.

Overall, the narratives of perpetrators born in the 1950s and 1960s—baby boomers, who grew up amid harsh political violence and unrest including dictatorships—often exhibited unapologetic language and a certain bravado in their descriptions of aggression. Furthermore, there were more references to social support, and a general indifference to the idea of being caught or framing their actions as wrong, indicating a more deeply entrenched discourse of impunity. These men, like Celso and Hugo, rationalised their violence as a means to re-establish control in their relationships, often justifying their actions as necessary responses to their partner's behaviour. Ultimately, their stories demonstrate a marked indifference to the consequences or moral implications of their actions.

Pears: New Stories, Milder Tales

"That day, what happened [slower tone] was just me being out of control. It was not, I will say as many times as I have to, not something I wanted to do." In this statement, Matías reflects on the murder he committed, highlighting a crucial distinction between generations of men convicted for this crime. From his narration, violence is something difficult to articulate without hesitation and, above all, something reprehensible. Like many men born between the 1980s and early 2000s, Matías draws on common narratives used to describe femicide: soap operas and newspapers began depicting such violence in more visible and complex ways in all the region. However, his approach sets him apart from his older counterparts: aggression, for him, is an action that demands justification, concealment, and a more complex explanation.

Younger perpetrators, like Matías, often frame their violent actions as *reactions to immediate emotional triggers*, with little reflection on the broader context or a longstanding pattern of behaviour. While they situate the femicide within the larger story of their intimate relationships, the narrative tends to narrow down to specific incidents, rather than being viewed as part of a wider, ongoing pattern. For example, one 29-year-old interviewee described his violent outburst as a result of feeling betrayed, stating, "She made me feel like I was nothing, and I just snapped." The rhetoric of snapping is a recurring one across generations, where violence is attributed to a sudden, overwhelming emotional trigger, often external to the relationship. Yet for Matías, as with other younger interviewees, this "snapping" is linked solely to the events immediately preceding the femicide. This way of telling the story rationalises the femicide by locating it within a particular situation, rather than seeing it as a product of broader relationship dynamics.

The expression of repentance varied significantly across generations. Younger perpetrators more often acknowledge the wrongfulness of their actions—framing them as regrettable yet 'logical' responses to specific provocations, such as feelings of betrayal or disrespect. Their remorse, though genuine, is frequently tempered by justifications rooted in the emotional intensity of the moment. In contrast, older men are less self-critical—focusing instead on regretting the consequences, such as negative outcomes or social fallout, rather than the violent act itself. They tend to justify their actions as necessary for restoring order or control, rarely questioning their legitimacy. While both generations may express regret for the aftermath—an issue beyond the scope of this book—younger men are more likely to acknowledge the harm caused, even as they rationalise it emotionally. Older men, however, often frame their violence within a broader, more calculated pattern of behaviour.

Finally, the language used by younger perpetrators is often *less blunt and vivid* in describing violence or coercive control. Unlike older men, who tend to use self-righteous, unapologetic language to justify their violence, younger men describe their actions with more emotional weight, emphasising the triggers that led to their violent outbursts. Expressions such as "I just snapped", "Didn't mean to", "Lost it completely", and "Couldn't think straight when I saw her" reflect this tendency. Overall, while both generations share similar narrative features, the way they tell their stories differs. This results in a greater effort to detach themselves from the violence as the focal point of their narratives.

From the "Killing" to the "Incident"

In an interview, a 34-year-old interviewee spoke strongly against a man in his early 60s, also incarcerated for femicide. "We might be in prison with the same *carátula* [charge sheet of the crime], but we are not the same type of man. He is heartless, he has no regrets. The way he talks about the crime…" While this man distanced himself from a specific individual in the same prison, likely in the context of numerous conflicts shaping his self-presentation, he made it clear: they do not tell their stories the same way.

Indeed, participants told their stories in different ways. When examining these narratives across different cohorts of men, contrasting elements became apparent. Most evidently, the language itself varied significantly. This reflects the vast differences in storytelling and slang across countries, cultures, and subcultures. Nonetheless, there is a consistent pattern: a shift in the words used. Younger men, for instance, increasingly relied on euphemisms, replacing terms like killing, murder, femicide, or even violence with softer alternatives such as incident, event, or moodiness. This shift may be seen as the result of a changing narrative landscape. Similarly, the roles of actors in their stories appeared to align with a different discursive context. The stark, binary portrayals of servile and master relationships common in older generations were no longer as straightforwardly depicted.

Bravado was also more pronounced in conversations with older men. Their accounts often featured blunt victim-blaming, with their rationalisations more explicitly defended. For younger interviewees, femicide was a more politically sensitive topic. Consequently, their storytelling tended to focus more on contextual or relational aspects that they perceived as mitigating factors. There was also a noticeable effort to erase traces of what could be described as intimate terrorism—the pattern of coercive control and sustained violence aimed at dominating and subjugating an intimate partner.

Younger interviewees also tended to provide less overt descriptions of aggression. This tendency reflects a broader shift in how violence is framed and narrated by younger people. Rather than openly describing acts of physical aggression, these individuals often downplayed or reframed their actions, opting for subtler language that minimised the intensity or intent of their behaviour. This could be connected to their heightened awareness of social norms and the stigma surrounding overt violence, particularly in contexts where politically correct discourse and sensitivity to gendered violence are more prominent. This reluctance to articulate aggression explicitly may also reflect an effort to distance themselves from the label of 'perpetrator', aligning their narratives with more socially acceptable or less incriminating portrayals.

Additionally, the justifications within their narratives—specific elements requiring explanation, elaboration, or contextualisation—shifted. The justifications offered by younger men reflected a more nuanced and complex effort to rationalise their actions. Unlike older cohorts, who might have relied on blunt victim-blaming or hierarchical notions of control, younger men's stories included more detailed contextual and relational elements. These elements were often framed as mitigating factors, such as misunderstandings, emotional states, or external pressures, which they believed could temper perceptions of culpability. The emphasis on these justifications indicates a shift in the narrative strategies employed, perhaps shaped by greater societal scrutiny of intimate partner violence and a growing awareness of the need to present their actions in a more defensible or sympathetic light. This evolution also underscores a change in how these men perceive the audience for their stories, tailoring their accounts to fit contemporary discursive expectations.

When considering the supporting narratives, it also becomes apparent that the mention of peer support became less explicit with time. While this was not a universal trend, the overall shift indicated that younger men were less likely to reference their peers when describing coercive control, seeking legitimation for violence, or even covering up abuse. This generational change in the narratives signalled an evolution in the repertoire of actors within these stories. While this may not necessarily reflect an actual variation in the networks involved in abuse, it does suggest a shifting 'scenography' in the way these stories are told.

This generational shift was also reflected in how men narrated their experiences with institutions and detection. Younger men described scenarios where institutional complicity—whether taking institutional support for granted or having the knowledge to circulate undetected while committing intimate partner violence—was notably less pervasive. Indeed, among the youngest participants, narratives that presumed the tacit approval of violence by others were almost entirely absent. Impunity featured far less as a backdrop in their accounts of more recent cases.

The fact that the fear of being *"manchado"* (stained) by a police report for battering was a significant concern for Alberto (born in the late 1970s), yet relegated to a mere anecdotal aside in Hugo's account (interviewed in his late 60s), exemplifies this generational shift. It is a contrast that not only marks a difference in experience but also signals a deeper transformation in how violence, accountability, and risk are narrated.

Shifting Regional Scenarios

With shifting narratives, an inevitable question emerges: why do differences arise in the storytelling of these cohorts? These changes, while not monumental, highlight consistent transformation in their stories. The sense of impunity, the implicit social support, the ease of victim-blaming, and the bravado with which aggression is described—all have evolved. Drawing on Jeff Hearn's (1998) classic framework, I argue that this transformation reflects a move from concession and revendication to a greater reliance on justifications and excuses.

Changes in discourse are undoubtedly complex, influenced by a multitude of factors that shape how stories are told. Narratives are inherently temporal, weaving together the past, present, and future (McKibben & Breheny, 2023). Stories about the past are inevitably shaped by the present context; when individuals recount an experience at a later time, their narratives are reframed by new insights gained through experience (Josselson, 2009). The non-linear, dynamic nature of narratives has been key to understanding the intersections of place, time, and identity. Considering this, the variations in the stories told by these men can be understood as arising from a combination of temporal and social aspects. These include the broader national social contexts and discursive frameworks that shape their narratives, the specific configurations of their local environments, the individual trajectories and narrative processes they undergo, and the influence of their prison experiences, including the length of their incarceration.

Another way to begin decoding differences in these narratives is to consider the context—and, most importantly, the narrative one—in which the men were born and raised. Acknowledging the social and political transformations that occurred may aid our interpretation of change. This is hardly a surprise, as dominant discourses are frequently the focal point of much scholarship dealing with biographies and gender-based violence (see Plummer, 2019; Rosenthal, 2010). The assumption here is that, as biographies are embedded in a specific context, changes in the contexts they traversed—and with which they interacted—will, in one way or another, lead to changes in the stories they tell.

Men born in the 1950s and 1960s came into the world during a time when Latin America was witnessing the growing stirrings of organised women's rights movements, influenced by both global trends and local political shifts. For instance, the expansion of women's suffrage marked significant milestones in countries such as Argentina (1947), Chile (1949), and Colombia (1957). This period also saw women increasingly participating in labour movements, particularly in urban centres where industrialisation created new employment opportunities (McGee Deutsch, 1991). For example, women in Brazil and Mexico began advocating for labour protections and equal pay.

These changes were part of what is often referred to as the second wave of feminism, which naturally carried regional nuances. As Espino (2024) describes, this period was characterised by intense political turmoil, with many countries experiencing military dictatorships, revolutionary movements, and widespread social unrest. For instance, Brazil underwent a coup in 1964, Chile faced political instability between 1964 and 1970 followed by a military takeover in 1973, and Uruguay was under military rule from 1973 to 1985. Feminist debates during this time in the region were not solely focused on gender inequality but also intertwined with broader political struggles for democracy, justice, and human rights (Barrancos, 2023). This dual focus often led to significant resistance against feminist mobilisations, with hardcore anti-feminist discourses actively pushing back—a phenomenon now commonly referred to as backlash, which expressed itself more severely in this context. Traditional gender roles remained deeply entrenched, with the idealisation of motherhood and domesticity continuing to dominate societal norms.

Men born during the 1970s and 1980s grew up amidst intense political upheaval, with military dictatorships and civil wars dominating much of the region. Despite—or perhaps because of—this instability, feminist movements gained momentum, often intersecting with broader struggles for democracy and human rights. The household became a central and contested space for political and gender-related debates (Johnson, 2000; Sapriza, 2015). In Argentina, the *Madres de Plaza de Mayo* emerged as a powerful symbol of resistance, as mothers of the disappeared demanded justice during the military dictatorship. Similarly, in Chile, women played a crucial role in grassroots organising against Pinochet's regime. These decades also saw the rise of feminist critiques of patriarchy and violence against women, leading to the first regional conferences on women's rights, such as the 1981 *Encuentro Feminista* in Bogotá. The fight for reproductive rights, including access to contraception and abortion, began to take shape, though progress was uneven across countries.

By the 1990s and early 2000s, many Latin American countries were undergoing democratic transitions, creating opportunities for the institutionalisation of gender equality initiatives. Governments established women's ministries and passed landmark legislation addressing gender-based violence, such as Brazil's Maria da Penha Law (2006) and Mexico's General Law on Women's Access to a Life Free of Violence (2007) (Pasinato & de Ávila, 2022). Gender quotas were introduced in politics, significantly increasing women's representation in legislatures across the region. For example, Argentina's 1991 Quota Law mandated that at least 30% of legislative candidates be women, inspiring similar reforms in neighbouring countries.

This period also witnessed the rise of grassroots feminist movements, culminating in campaigns like *Ni Una Menos*, which began in Argentina in 2015 and quickly spread across the region. *Ni Una Menos* protests highlighted the 'epidemic of femicide' and gender-based violence, mobilising millions of women and allies. Additionally, the global #MeToo movement resonated in Latin America, amplifying conversations about workplace harassment and sexual violence. These movements revitalised the push for reproductive rights, leading to historic victories such as the legalisation of abortion in Argentina in 2020 and the decriminalisation of abortion in Mexico in 2023. Despite these achievements, backlash from conservative sectors, particularly the Catholic Church and evangelical movements, underscore the ongoing struggle for gender equality in the region.

Eroding Gendered Recipes?

> Hence we no longer perceive the same things as real, and coincident with our vanishing sense of a common reality we are losing our common medium for expressing and communicating our experiences. The world has been splintered into countless fragments of atomized individuals and groups. The disruption in the wholeness of individual experience corresponds to the disintegration in culture and group solidarity. When the bases of unified collective action begin to weaken, the social structure tends to break. (Mannheim, 1991, p. XXV)

Much like Mannheim's observation about generational change, connecting individual stories with changing macro-social structures offers valuable insights into why these narratives evolve. The shifting socio-political contexts in which perpetrators were born and raised provide a useful framework for understanding how men from different generations tend to narrate their stories in distinct ways. Despite the diverse national nuances, evolving discourses around gender, women's rights, and men's roles may ultimately point in the same direction. This empirical observation invites several interpretations, highlighting the intersection of personal experiences with broader social transformations.

One thesis is to view change as the *weakening of a dominant narrative*: specifically, the gradual erosion of male-chauvinist scripts resulting from decades of social mobilisation and the eventual integration (and, at times, co-option) of the fight against gender violence into state policies. The shift in how blunt and self-assured the younger men appear in their narratives suggests their struggle with the residual cultural baggage of earlier generations and entrenched structures. This perspective points to a steady decline in the legitimacy of discourses that normalise this form of violence, potentially aligning with the observed, albeit slow, decrease in femicide rates over recent decades (UNODC & UN Women, 2024). In essence, this interpretation frames social change as a cumulative legacy of layered transformations.

This reading of narrative weakening aligns with Maristella Svampa's (2000) concept of "splintered identities" (*identidades astilladas*). Originally introduced to critique how shifts in political and economic regimes fragment once-cohesive institutionalised labour identities, this concept provides a useful lens for understanding how transformations in the social fabric—encompassing both dominant discourses and tangible social relationships—destabilise traditional masculine identities. From this perspective, the interviews within this cohort reveal how men's storytelling is shaped by distinct historical processes. These shifting, temporally bound narratives underscore the fragmentation of once-dominant scripts. While these fractured narratives may appear less overtly harmful, they remain damaging, manifesting in subtler and less visible ways, untethered from a singular, mainstream master narrative.

Alternatively, this phenomenon could be interpreted as the *delegitimisation of these narratives in public discourse*, prompting men to express them less openly. This could be seen as a form of situational adaptation, where such narratives are downplayed in face-to-face interactions or articulated less explicitly in general. Here, the focus lies on the narrative performance (Labov & Waletzky, 1997): the virtual persona presented to an audience (such as an interviewer), and not on the identity itself. This perspective may align with the observation that, despite fluctuations and a slight decline, femicide rates in Latin America have remained relatively stable over the last decade.

Although these interpretations are presented separately, they are not necessarily contradictory. Nor should these changes be dismissed as inconsequential. The shifting dynamics in masculinities and the destabilisation of traditional gender regimes, point to small dislocations within societal structures. For example, Gottzén's (2019) concept of "chafing masculinity" highlights the discomfort and shame associated with certain sexist practices, signalling their delegitimisation, while also acknowledging the slow-paced identity changes involved. The evolving narratives may be driven by these shifts in identities and the emergence of new repertoires for telling these stories. Here, contradiction is not an obstacle to understanding this phenomenon; rather, it reflects the complexity and depth of unconscious processes (Sinclair & Steinkoler, 2018).

The limited availability of therapeutic interventions for perpetrators, coupled with the persistence of penal states, warrants consideration alongside these interpretations. In the vast majority of the institutions where the interviews took place, there are no treatment programmes (psychological, psychiatric, or counselling sessions), meaning there was less active involvement in the reshaping of their narratives. In certain cases, like Alberto's, participation in masculinity programmes occurred more by chance than as part of a deliberate strategy of state institutions. This scarcity of intervention underscores the necessity of addressing these narratives within comprehensive support frameworks post-incarceration.

Ultimately, young perpetrators are likely to be released from prison in their mid-40s and still have future partners. Our collective disengagement with this fact signals that we are not fully considering the urgent need for early interventions and the development of comprehensive support systems. These should not only focus on the time spent in prison but also on the long-term 'reintegration' of these men into society, where their narratives and behaviours can be reshaped in healthier directions. Yet, a paradox remains: can we truly 'reintegrate' perpetrators back *into* a patriarchal society?

This chapter does not aim to provide a definitive answer to the question of how femicide narratives change over time or their connection to femicide rates. Given the virtual absence of research and discussion on this issue, its purpose is to spark a conversation as well as a theoretical exploration. While current discussions in the field focus, for instance, on reimagining femicide measurements (e.g., Walklate & Fitz-Gibbon, 2023) and on alternative epistemological approaches to femicide data (D'Ignazio, 2024), we still struggle to address and discuss the evolving logics of perpetrators and, in this case, how we can understand their transformation.

10

What If...? A Counterfactual Experiment

> Outside the reference books, I had personally collected the details of a hundred and eighty cases, all downloaded from the judicial records [...]. Professions of the accused: soldier, electrician, builder's mate, farm labourer, civil servant, student. You could say that some killing is a democratic sort of crime. (Melo, 2023, p. 14)

A Gender-Swapping Breaching Experiment

In *Gender Swapped Fairy Tales* (2021), Fransman and Plackett cleverly explore how dominant gender narratives function by reversing the genders of protagonists in classic fairy tales (Fig. 10.1). This device exposes some deep-seated assumptions that shape these stories, such as characters in distress, heroic arcs of overcoming evil, and gendered traits like women being nurturing or men as rescuers. By swapping the genders, these rigid frameworks become more evident, highlighting how profoundly they structure our worldview. A locked-up Mr Rapunzel in a tower feels jarringly out of place, while a fragile Handsome seems almost

M. H. Di Marco, *Narratives of Femicide Perpetrators in Latin America*, https://doi.org/10.1007/978-3-031-97367-3_10

too 'modern' in his dynamic with the Beast. Even when these tales are retold with innovative twists, the persistent underlying narratives create a sense of dissonance.

The same principle applies to the stories perpetrators tell. These narratives reproduce societal scripts, consciously or unconsciously, even when they appear to challenge or diverge from them. Such stories can reflect entrenched expectations about masculinity, dominance, and control, just as fairy tales mirror cultural ideals of femininity and heroism. By examining these patterns, we gain a clearer understanding of how narratives—whether in fairy tales or personal accounts—serve as vehicles for broader social norms.

The narratives condensed in this book—arguably as archetypal as fairy tales in their portrayal through media, novels, and shows—invite similar questions. What would happen if we reversed the genders in their stories? Would the narrative remain equally compelling? Although a counterfactual exercise, it may help expose that these stories operate within a broader social framework than is often assumed. In essence, this experiment aims to test whether these swapped narratives would remain logical and coherent, or whether they would collapse into absurdity.

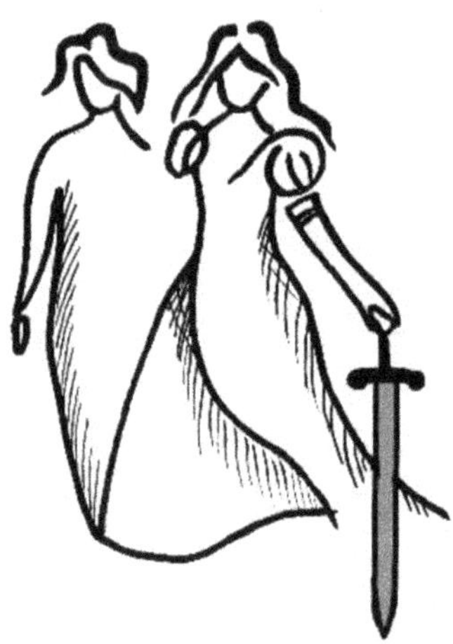

Fig. 10.1 Swapping genders

Inspired by Fransman and Plackett's approach, this chapter presents an ad hoc experiment aimed at exploring the scope of the narrative. While working on the manuscript, I explored a twofold strategic alteration of the vignettes: in one case, I swapped the genders of the protagonists, and in another, I replaced the femicide with a 'heated' fight, without the use of physical violence. I specifically did this with the first five vignettes presented here.

With this approach, Jorge (Chapter 6.1) became Celina. The reimagined story depicted a woman who grew increasingly insecure about her boyfriend studying and making new friends. Her mounting anxieties escalated to the point where he no longer baked her favourite birthday cake for her special day. "Only God knows why I got so excited about my birthdays. But I never wanted anything too extravagant—just the simple things in life. A nice party, a good meal, a birthday cake. And he knew that. We spent many birthdays together, and he knew. I remember asking him for a cake I loved when we were first dating because I knew he was a fantastic baker." For João (Chapter 6.3), the story retained the same gender of the protagonists, but physical violence and the brutal murder were replaced with frequent, intense arguments: "The night shifts were a bloody nightmare because we were knackered the next day. We never got much sleep, were in a foul mood, and utterly exhausted, so we started blowing all our money on weed. It was only natural that we started arguing. We were in a right strop all day long."

Nineteen Latin American male scholars from the social, human, and mainly medical sciences read drafts of the vignettes during a general workshop on qualitative methodology, all of whom were unfamiliar with my work and the book's central argument. That all participants were men—and engaged in this discussion—was a fortunate coincidence, one that later evolved into a fruitful conversation about gender and storytelling within the workshop.

I posed three questions to the readers, seeking to uncover different aspects of their responses to the altered stories. The first question, *How did you find the overall story?*, was intended to capture the reader's initial reaction to the narrative. The second, *How unusual or extraordinary were the scenarios and situations described?*, sought to determine whether the altered scenarios felt unconventional or deviated from the reader's expectations. The final question, *Did the storylines seem fitting?*, aimed to assess whether the plot and characters' actions appeared logical and coherent given the gender reversal or the ending of the stories.

During a subsequent meeting in this workshop, I clarified the original motive behind my writing, noting that I had deliberately altered the vignettes. This clarification led to an in-depth conversation about narratives and their structures and the impact on interpretations that people have.

This experience was heavily inspired by Garfinkel's (1967) famous breaching experiment, which deliberately disrupts social norms or expectations to observe how people respond and attempt to restore order. For instance, speaking loudly in a library challenges the implicit expectation of silence, prompting reactions that reveal how norms are maintained in everyday interactions. Indexicality plays a key role in this process, as individuals rely on contextual cues to interpret meaning and preserve coherence. When these cues are disrupted, familiar frameworks become difficult to apply, prompting people to recontextualise the situation in an attempt to make sense of it within their existing cognitive and cultural schemas. In this case, altering the narratives and asking readers to interpret the stories functions as a breaching experiment, challenging entrenched assumptions about gender roles and crime. By unsettling these norms, the experiment exposes how deeply they influence perception and interpretation.

Unindexed Narratives

Surprisingly, the feedback was more varied than I had anticipated. The responses to the altered vignettes were far from uniform: for most readers, something felt 'off', making the narratives seem less plausible. However, for others, particularly when reading the versions where arguments replaced femicides, the script appeared comprehensible and, in some cases, even relatable. These reactions, presented here in an archetypal manner, reveal narratives much like an X-ray, bringing to light the underlying structures that shape familiar stories.

Odd Storylines: 'What?!' Interpretations

Some readers immediately sensed that something was amiss in the texts. They found the events and their presentation inconsistent—as though the pieces did not quite fit together. Some even regarded them as absurd. This reaction typically arose when the stories were gender-swapped while the murders remained unchanged. The roles assigned to female perpetrators and male victims seemed misplaced, leading these readers to perceive the plot as unrealistic or overly exaggerated. The men's alleged infidelity, the women's violent reactions 'out of passion', and their attempts to control their male partners were sometimes even described with humour by the readers. This reaction reveals an important insight: the male-perpetrator plot was the familiar trope. More significantly, the actions of male perpetrators were more readily understood and, to some extent, excused.

Faced with this unsettling sense of dissonance, readers sought to resolve the discrepancy by assuming that something was wrong with the plot or that a crucial piece of information was missing. As they attempted to reconcile this breach of expectation, questions emerged: for Celina (in the swapped case of Jorge, Chapter 6.1), a participant asked "Why would a girlfriend be so obsessed with making her boyfriend bake a birthday cake?"; for Liza (in Celso's adapted case, Chapter 6.2), another one interrogated "What kind of friendships would a woman need to ask her friends for such things?"; and for Josefa (in the swapped Héctor case, Chapter 6.3), another participant claimed, "It seems too simplistic that she would be so obsessed with her husband returning to work after being a homemaker. Something doesn't add up."

Evidently, the familiar arcs of male aggressors and female victims had been disrupted, and the new roles seemed misaligned with their cultural understanding of gender norms. A storyline in which a woman committed violence against a man felt jarring and unnatural, making the plot seem disjointed and difficult to believe. Their responses underscored how much our expectations of a logical narrative depend on gendered scripts. This tension between what is presented and the expectations of the audience exposed how ingrained they were in a specific gendered framing of violence. When a woman killed her male partner over something as trivial as failing to bake a cake, it shattered not only their understanding of gender but also their conceptions of violence itself.

Either finding these stories unrealistic or outright absurd, readers' immediate reactions were telling. The narratives did not follow the expected arcs that readers are predominantly exposed to—making their responses entirely understandable. This was a key point of the experiment: if readers found it strange for a woman to state, "She was not a jealous woman; he made her jealous [on purpose]" (based on swapped Celso), it suggested the presence of an underlying narrative shaping our cognition—where the inverted situation seemed more plausible. The stories did not 'fit the mould'—leading readers to question the plausibility of the events.

Comprehensible Storylines: 'I Get It' Interpretations

A different dynamic emerged when the narratives retained the genders of the characters but replaced the femicide with a 'strong discussion'. Despite some reservations, readers generally found the stories logical. Despite some reservations, readers generally found the stories coherent. This contrasted sharply with how the same actions were interpreted by readers of the original vignettes—and potentially how they would have been interpreted had the gender roles been reversed. In these cases, conflict and aggression appeared to 'fit' within emotional and relational norms typically attributed to men, even though the same justifications would not apply in the opposite scenario. One workshop participant remarked, "Well, I think I would react the same way if she cheated on me, to be frank."

Overall, when the protagonist engaged in non-physical violence—such as Celina-Jorge feeling hurt when her partner did not bake a cake, or Helena-Héctor opposing her husband returning to work after decades as a homemaker—readers tended to perceive their actions as more understandable, even excusable. In most cases, they justified the anger and controlling behaviour as a response to emotional turmoil, often linked to betrayal, strain, or extenuating circumstances. These behaviours were framed within emotional, relational, or gendered norms that legitimised such responses—norms that would not apply if the genders were reversed.

As a narrative response, 'I get it' essentially meant that readers deemed the described scenario comprehensible and, in some cases, relatable. This suggested that the events were acknowledged as not only expectable but even anticipated. In particular, supporting friendships in 'dire' personal situations, finding difficulty adapting to a partner's renewed desire to return to work after decades, and generally confronting the feeling of being left were also justified.

To understand this interpretation labour by the readers, highlighting the active role of emotions is fruitful. Empathy—or more appropriately himpathy (Manne, 2017)—played a key role in shaping these interpretations. It functioned as a device to render the narratives comprehensible and, more importantly, to provide a moral evaluation. One way in which himpathy operated was through assumed situational factors that rationalised the violence: "Perhaps alcohol or drugs were involved", or "Everyone has bad moments in their lives." Others drew on personal experiences to soften their explanations of the stories.

This active interpretation of the readers underscores the deeply rooted double standards in how male and female aggression is viewed, especially in intimate partner violence. It points to the way dominant cultural narratives can shape the way we understand and justify conflict, aggression and peer support depending on who is perpetrating them. The experiment highlighted how gendered perceptions influence the moral and emotional framing of violent acts, with male protagonists often receiving more empathy or less condemnation in comparison to female perpetrators when men read this stories. Our interpretive frameworks are not as neutral as we like to believe, and that gender assumptions significantly affect how we engage with stories of violence.

Putting Us in the Picture

> You have to leave the island in order to see the island, that we can't see ourselves unless we become free of ourselves. (Saramago, 2000, p. 20)

The main aim of this experiment was to extend our understanding of these narratives beyond the niche context of femicide perpetrators and explore how they resonated with other cisgender men. Potentially, a similar argument could be made for women and diversities as well. The underlying assumption is that we tend to conceptualise femicide—and violence more broadly—through a rapid process of othering: perpetrators ultimately become 'bad apples'. This creates a division, with nothing connecting 'us' with 'them'. When it comes to reprehensible actions, distancing ourselves from aggressors serves not only to establish a symbolic yet reassuring barrier—convincing us that we do not share the same traits as those deemed 'outliers' or 'monsters'—but also to obscure the social conditions that enable such violence in the first place.

I am particularly interested in resisting the impulse to other, primarily because it relies heavily on the privilege of distance—a perspective that not only normalises and simplifies punishment but also forecloses the possibility of envisioning alternative legal systems and mechanisms for social change (Brown, 2013; Shuman, 2010). While it is undoubtedly true that these men have committed a particularly heinous act that most people have not, framing their worldviews as entirely alien to ours denies the social nature of femicide—it is, ultimately, a social product. Both of the narrative responses to the modified vignettes illustrate how such narratives circulate widely. The 'what?!' (demonstrating narrative dissonance) and 'I get it' (showing plausibility alignment) reactions point to the same implicit norms. In short, this breaching experiment highlights the dangers of othering violence: this manoeuvre detaches it from the very system that produces and sustains it.

We can largely interpret plausibility alignment—when the familiar stories we have heard and internalised shape how we make sense of new ones—as an embodied reflection of society's complicity in gendered hierarchies. In the end, "if misogyny seeks to punish women who challenge gendered hierarchies, himpathy functions as its protective counterpart, offering moral cover for those who enforce these hierarchies" (Manne, 2017, p. 37). Those engaging with these narratives are not merely analysing gender—they are feeling it, just as the perpetrators and their male friends do. They link these stories to their past experiences, connecting them with bodily emotions (hurt, passion, anger), making this alignment a deeply embedded, subterranean process rather than a purely cognitive one. We are inevitably all deeply invested in gendered social hierarchies: we have something at stake in them.

It should become evident that these narratives were not unique to the men interviewed. Instead, the exercise revealed that sexist narratives about intimate relationships, expectations, conflicts, and disruption of the status quo are far more pervasive. Kate Manne captures this point so powerfully—bringing the collective 'us' into the discussion—that I find it fitting to quote her directly. In *Down Girl* (2017, p. XXI), she eloquently writes:

> I belabour the point because I believe that, in much of our thinking and acting, we channel and enact social forces far beyond our threshold of conscious awareness or even ability to recover—and sometimes, markedly contrary to our explicit moral beliefs and political commitments. There is hence a risk of convincing ourselves, on the basis of post hoc reasoning, not to look too hard at the residual patriarchal forces operating in our culture, as the patriarchal forces themselves gather in the backroom to laugh at our expense and grow stronger in our absence. In my grimmer moods, I picture party hats and hooters.

Patriarchal forces persist and flourish—often unnoticed—within the fabric of our cultural and personal lives, and should not be understood as existing outside of us (there is no "backroom"). Including ourselves and our imaginaries in the discussion may be fruitful not only to avoid the sometimes futile othering of those who cause harm but also because othering obscures the structural nature of the problem in the first place. As narratives become "sticky", they embed themselves in our embodied experiences, shaping our feelings, actions, and views in ways that influence our perceptions and interactions (Ahmed, 2004). We are part of the equation. This involvement extends not only to us as 'listeners' of these stories but also as interpreters and reproducers of these narratives. Even the fact that we might find these swapped stories absurd would highlight how dominant stories affect us as well, demonstrating the narrative power they hold in shaping our understanding of gender.

Acknowledging that others play a role in the reproduction of these narratives, and incorporating that reasoning into our critique, offers a much-needed perspective on the role of the social sciences, particularly criminology. Expanding our understanding of stories—dislocating them from perpetrators alone—can help counteract the passive, voyeuristic engagement with punishment or penal spectatorship (Bunn, 2023) and the portrayal of the 'criminal' as an abject subject, contrasted with a non-criminal suspended in the abstract. This would not only expose how social sciences can be complicit in voyeuristic practices that reinforce exclusion but also underscore the need for a broader, more encompassing perspective.

We often assume that the circulation and reproduction of narratives originate from centralised power structures—an abstract entity termed patriarchy—or formal institutions such as schools and the media (Plummer, 2019). However, face-to-face interactions might be placed at the centre of our discussion and analytical focus. These exchanges do not merely reinforce dominant narratives but reveal a web of coexisting and competing discourses. My argument here is that these are not distinct narratives. These are not stories told exclusively by femicide perpetrators (except for the killing itself). Rather, they are widely available scripts. Logically, they extend beyond these men and circulate—likely with varying degrees of adherence and intensity—throughout social spaces. A brief look at fictional narratives or even academic scholarship reveals similar themes. The question remains, however: what makes these narratives end in fatality for some, and not for others?

11

Conclusions

Thinking Back

This book set out to address central, yet often taken for granted, questions about men convicted of intimate femicide in Latin America: What stories do they tell to give meaning to this crime? What underlying layers of meaning are present in these stories, and how do they shift over time? And are there similar patterns of interpretation across the region that reveal the power of these narratives?

In a radical artistic way, *The House That Jack Built* (the controversial 2018 film directed by Lars von Trier) offers an exploration of the psyche of a serial killer through the life of Jack, a disturbed and obsessive individual. The film unfolds with Jack recounting 12 of his murders of women. However, it is only in the closing scenes that the narrator, Virgil, confronts Jack, asking, "Did you realise you describe all the women as stupid?" Throughout the story, female characters are portrayed as weak, gullible, and naïve, existing primarily to fulfil Jack's sadistic desires. This portrayal is subtly veiled until the film's conclusion, demonstrating the filmmaker's skill in masking this critique from the audience. It is only then that viewers are compelled to confront Jack's misogynistic descriptions of women.

M. H. Di Marco, *Narratives of Femicide Perpetrators in Latin America*,
https://doi.org/10.1007/978-3-031-97367-3_11

Similarly, the narratives that underpin intimate femicides, as examined in this book, largely operate beneath the surface, embedded within cultural frameworks and embodied stories. The stories of these men, once obscured, are brought to light through the legal proceedings involving the interviewed men (when the code femicide or feminicide is put into practice) and subsequently through the interview process, which raises questions that uncover a multitude of meanings. As Geertz (1973) famously argued, it is only by treating culture as a text—something that can be read and analysed—that we can objectify its underlying meanings. This, however, remains an inherently imperfect endeavour.

Unlike von Trier's portrayal of a misogynistic mind, interviewing real men presents a series of challenges. We do not have a reflective an almost omniscient narrator, like Virgil, to guide our questions, nor is there a universally recognisable 'evil core' within the souls of these individuals. Moreover, the veracity of their stories might become a central concern for some analysts. However, while there may not always be a Machiavellian rationale behind every account, socio-cultural contexts undeniably shape these events—though these influences can be difficult to delineate. Gender norms, in particular, become a significant part of this equation.

The twentieth century witnessed numerous successful efforts to advance the study of perpetrators and their stories across various fields (Feld & Salvi, 2019; Hearn, 1998; Robben & Hinton, 2023). However, when it comes to examining extreme violence such as femicide or sexual violence, a gap in research remains (Evans et al., 2023; Kruse & Skilbrei, 2024). Much of the prevailing scholarship on femicide perpetrators still tends to adopt an individualising perspective or rely on overly reductionist, structuralist frameworks that portray perpetrators as mere automatons of patriarchy.

It should be evident that understanding femicide perpetration is an exceedingly complex endeavour. One dimension of this crime involves exploring the motives as articulated and recorded in judicial terms—what legal discourse translates and determines. Another dimension considers the unconscious psychological elements tied to desire and the act itself, as forensic and legal psychology might examine. Yet another perspective views femicide as a byproduct of shared narratives within society that enable such acts—a socio-narrative approach. This latter path, adopted in this book, aims to reconnect individual murders to the broader structural phenomenon of violence against women.

While meaning is central to all these questions, the way it is approached varies significantly. This book began with the premise that issues of meaning and intention render certain quests for answers inherently fraught, if not doomed to failure. At the heart of this complexity—and the book's aim—is the definition itself: the killing of a woman or girl 'on account of her gender'. The latest UNODC & UN Women report (2024), for instance, underscores this, stating:

> Motives are rooted in societal norms and stereotypes that consider women to be subordinate to men, as well as in discrimination towards women and girls, inequality, and unequal power relations between women and men in society. (p. 10)

Recapitulation

This book explores the perpetration of femicide through three main analytical aims. It highlighted how the ways we organise meaning and engage with socially available frameworks—essentially the learned stories about events, actors, roles, and so on—play a crucial role in fostering femicide. Understanding these structures not only sheds light on the meanings surrounding gender, relationships, and harm—often oversimplified in mainstream discourses—but also reveals the expectations these men held, the 'irreversible' turning points in their stories, and how their stories intertwined to devastating effect. Additionally, this work engages with a fundamental assumption in social science: that to understand violence, we cannot take its performance for granted. This paradox of violence—our reluctance to engage with 'heinous' criminals, as Riches (1986) described—limits our understanding. Finally, the book deconstructs broad terms like 'healthy son of patriarchy' and machismo, which, while commonly used, have become reified. As with any dominant interpretive schema, these terms can obscure as much as they reveal when they are applied without critical reflection (Bandelli, 2017). Once any discourse becomes *doxa*—when we stop questioning it—it becomes difficult to recognise the mechanisms it uses to shape our worlds.

Through the use of vignettes, I establish five arguments. A shared narrative element in the stories of these men across Latin America is rule-breaking. Lethal violence may be framed in various ways—such as sudden, as the culmination of bidirectional violence, or as a calculated action—yet the common thread is that violence was instrumentally used to punish and uphold a moral norm. The disruption of an expectation serves as the key turning point in these stories, where control emerges as a strategy to preserve a particular scenario. Violence is, thus, perceived and presented as a righteous action, creating a situation in which murder might not be framed as the central problem of the story. Narratives framing violence in this way were consistently shared by these men across the region.

A second argument is that femicide narratives are often accompanied by a range of supporting stories focused on non-intimate social relationships. These stories may be broader (e.g., those related to friendship, institutional reliability, and fragility), but they all converge to the point where the femicide narrative cannot be fully understood without them. In particular, stories about male peers supporting violence and impunity, where acquaintances are portrayed as passive witnesses and institutions are easily navigated for personal gain, are central. In some cases, there are stories of actors enabling, protecting, or fostering violence through a "himpathetic social system" (Manne, 2017, p. 45). This argument underscores that, without a broader perspective on these narratives—including networks of complicity, the taken-for-granted impunity operating behind these rationalities, and institutional inaction—these stories may lack practical significance. I find this argument to be the most relevant contribution of the book to the current discussion of femicide and the effort to prevent it.

A third argument in the book is that, even in extreme cases where the language of perpetrators takes on an unusual form—such as being disorganised or lacking expected elements like remorse—traces of narrative structures remain, providing a framework to make sense of the crimes. While extreme cases might invite the application of readily accessible psychological labels, such as psychopathy, it is evident that socially embedded discourses continue to shape and influence these men's accounts and guiding their actions. Furthermore, the ways in which perpetrators weave contextual elements into their stories vary, offering situational interpretations of their perspectives. Despite these differences, their narratives consistently reveal underlying contextual coordinates and deeply ingrained misogyny.

A fourth argument revolves around generational change among perpetrators in Latin America. The exploratory question—aimed more at fostering a much-needed discussion about the future than at providing a definitive answer about change—is what insights variations in 'narrative voice' offer about the historical moment we are navigating. While core elements, such as the safeguarding of moral norms, have remained consistent, younger perpetrators told stories with a reduced sense of impunity, less implicit social support, diminished victim-blaming, and a decline in the bravado with which aggression is described. This shift can be seen as a movement from concession and revendication to a greater reliance on justifications and excuses (Hearn, 1998). Comparing the stories of men born in the 1950s and 1960s—who experienced the early stirrings of organised women's rights movements, such as suffrage and the push for women to enter the workforce, alongside parallel dictatorships and patriarchal backlash—with those of men born in the 1990s and early 2000s—when feminist ideas and human rights logic had gradually been incorporated into states and daily life, albeit not without resistance—reveals this transformation.

This change could be interpreted as the weakening of a dominant narrative, specifically the gradual erosion of male-chauvinist stories resulting from decades of social mobilisation and eventual integration. Alternatively, it could be seen as the delegitimisation of these narratives in public discourse, leading men to express them less openly. Regardless of the interpretation, the changing pattern in storytelling (whether observed on a structural scale or in face-to-face interactional rules) should be recognised as a sign of a shifting narrative landscape and, hopefully, a positive transformation that aligns with declining rates of femicide.

A final argument in this chapter emerges from a breaching experiment in which vignettes were altered—either through gender swapping or replacing murder with a non-physical argument—and then discussed with an audience unfamiliar with the topic. This experiment challenges the impulse to 'other' perpetrators by revealing how these narratives align with entrenched gendered expectations and power dynamics, even among those not directly involved. Rather than viewing femicide as an act detached from social structures, I argue that misogynistic stories and himpathetic efforts should be recognised as pervasive, cross-cutting forces within society. By acknowledging the widespread nature of these narratives, I call for a shift in how we engage with and critique these stories, urging a more inclusive perspective that resists voyeuristic or punitive frameworks and, instead, explores the social conditions that sustain these harmful narratives.

All in all, the message weaving these arguments together is that for femicide to occur, a narrative must sustain its performance. For this to happen, the narrative focused on women and intimate relationships must be complemented by stories that justify violence, instil trust in impunity, and garner social support. Without these stories about institutions, friendships, kinship, and societal structures, femicide is difficult to comprehend as a social act. Without these stories, risk factors are scarcely understandable. Without these stories, upstream policies are difficult to conceptualise.

Narrative Hubs

"Si te agarro con otro te mato,
Te doy una paliza y después me escapo.
Dicen que yo soy violento,
Pero no te olvides que yo no soy lento.
Dicen que soy absorbente,
Porque siempre quiero tenerte presente.
Dicen que soy aburrido
Porque no me gusta que tengas amigos,
Que llegan de madrugada,
Y como son amigos, que no pasa nada."

"If I catch you with another, I'll kill you,

I'll give you a beating and then I'll flee.
They say I'm violent,
But don't forget, I'm not slow.
They say I'm possessive,
Because I always want you with me.
They say I'm boring,
Because I don't like you having friends,
Who show up at dawn,
And since they're friends, it's supposed to mean nothing."
(Cacho Castaña, Si te agarro con otro te mato).

The lyrics of *Si te agarro con otro te mato* (If I Find You with Another Man, I'll Kill You), performed by the Argentine bolero singer Cacho Castaña, offer a striking example of how love, violence, and control can be framed in a positive light—as part of folk romance—within a specific cultural and historical context. Released in 2003, the song's storyline might now be recognised by readers of this book as an overt manifestation of misogyny and even an apology for violence against women. However, even now, many listeners may interpret it more as a symbol of romance than of violence. Beyond serving as an illustrative example of such narratives, the song also underscores the production and dissemination of these stories within narrative hubs.

The question of the circulation of narratives raises a significant question to understand any form of violence: where are these narratives socialised, adapted, and reproduced? And how are they instilled? As Plummer (2019) argues, narrative hubs of engagement have a fundamental role as they function as mechanisms of social control: they regulate our interpretations and actions in society. The stories told by perpetrators are, in this sense, dual in nature: while they may be deeply personal accounts, often crafted to rationalise and persuade an audience, they also function as instruments of cultural power. Attention must therefore be directed towards the origins of these narratives.

Stories are not merely told; they are selected, shaped, supported, rewarded and 'tolerated' by the institutions to which we are committed and within which we live. This echoes Bruner's (2002) argument that institutions such as law, psychiatry, medicine, government, and education create and rely on specific ways of narrating human events. Media, books, and schools, for instance, play a key role in producing and perpetuating these narratives. Plummer (2019) also highlights an often-overlooked aspect in narrative research: the sources of dialogic narrative power. Beyond institutional, communicative, and locational sources, everyday interactions—such as face-to-face encounters or the social environments of schools—help shape the stories that emerge within the power dynamics of daily life.

Therefore, focusing on narrative hubs—or the sources that prominently amplify certain rationalities—inevitably leaves other practical projects addressing femicide somewhat exposed. For instance, the judicial system primarily tackles individual cases with punitive actions, as restorative justice in femicide and gender-based violence has yet to gain significant traction.

The peril we face today in the endeavour to understand and dismantle these misogynistic hubs is that, despite significant social movements and transformative efforts, we may claim victory too soon. Narratives that foster violence are far from exotic or rare. This is compounded by three common fallacies. There is an assumption of universal ease in diagnosing violence and aggression, coupled with the mistaken belief in a shared understanding of what constitutes violence. As Rose (2021) aptly notes, "It is a truism to say that everyone knows violence when they see it, but if one thing has become clear over the past decade, it is that the most prevalent, insidious forms of violence are those that cannot be easily seen" (p. 1).

Additionally, there is an assumption about the emotions involved in violence: 'violence is about badly managed repressed anger' or 'violence is a result of poor impulse control'. In my view, this is even more obscured, as it gives the impression of adopting a progressive critical lens while, in fact, it may merely reproduce politically correct naïve ideas of violence. As hooks (2004) argues, patriarchy primarily values anger when expressed by men: "Real men get mad. [...] Anger is the best hiding place for anybody seeking to conceal pain or anguish of spirit" (p. 22). Blaming anger or a lack of emotional skills has become an easily accessible explanation of violence, but it only superficially explains perpetration. Moreover, it overlooks the broader reality of the limited or nascent public discourse on emotions and frustration.

Finally, there is a fixation on the existence of single narrative as the unidimensional 'alpha and omega' of femicide. The critical question I pose to this approach is: are narratives about intimate relationships disconnected from broader ones tied to conflict and emotional turmoil? What about institutional reliability? Are these narratives complemented by how we make sense of conflicts more generally? For example, can we address the emotional illiteracy of perpetrators without understanding their everyday lives? It is not simply that "they lack the cognitive resources to…" but rather that this is a logical consequence of the patriarchal political economy's disinterest in fostering such skills. Emotional illiteracy is ultimately a product of social structures and not easily remedied by psychotherapy alone. This critique may provide not only contextual depth to our understanding but also more resources to work with.

If risk factors help identify features that play a specific role in fostering risk, reconnecting narratives into tessellations (for instance, connecting our stories of violence and friendship support) serves to identify the connective tissue between these scripts. Tessellations, in this sense, represent the opposite hermeneutic manoeuvre to individualisation: rather than assuming individual features contribute to the phenomenon, they suggest the phenomenon emerges from these connections themselves.

Inevitably, the approach of this book leans towards a broad-strokes understanding of femicide in Latin America and its hubs. As argued throughout, the main argument involves identifying the common narratives underpinning these stories across different times and places in the region. This is, above all, an introduction to many of the issues it raises. While the book delves into the life stories of men, its ultimate interest lies in how these accounts are products not only of situated agents but also of collective actions repeated over time and through hubs of engagement. I argue that a shared narrative economy fosters these killings, with recognisable structures evident across many Latin American countries. Furthermore, I contend that these narratives are interdependent with others, such as those of social support, complicity, and institutional impunity.

These discussions hopefully open the door for a deeper exploration of these narratives and their circulation within our societies. Certainly, social class, ethnicity, and specific positionalities can provide further nuance to our understanding of these stories, just as the particular social context may shape not only the reception but also the specific uses and effects of these narratives. In any case, this creates an opportunity to more specifically comprehend this narrative landscape and its hubs.

Thinking Ahead

> Individually and collectively, we need stories. It is a universal impulse. We need some galvanising, sense-making framework, a narrative, in order to instil order and a sense of purpose to our lives. Some myths are not only useful, they are necessary. All political orders are based on useful fictions which have allowed groups of humans, from ancient Mesopotamia through to the Roman empire and modern capitalist societies, to cooperate in numbers far beyond the scope of any other species. Every social unit, from the family to the nation state, functions on the basis of mythology, stories that set them apart from others. (Malik, 2019, p. 3)

I would argue that working with violence places us in a particularly unique position regarding our ethical understanding of knowledge production. It compels us, one way or another, to reflect on the usefulness of our enterprise, the autonomy of the academic agenda, and the practical implications we are—or are not—developing in our projects. My perspective, after writing this book, strongly resonates with the classic 11th thesis on Feuerbach: *"The philosophers have only interpreted the world, in various ways; the point is to change it"* (Mark, 1969 [1845], p. 14).

If we have learned certain narratives, we can learn new ones. Change, however, is far from a unilinear process; it is multifaceted and cannot be achieved through normative planning. When we specifically discuss narrative change, some aspects stand out. From the onset, change directly affects a network of individuals, institutions, policies, and, most importantly, traditions that are often resistant to alterations in status quo. These narratives are not merely articulated by powerful individuals on their platforms but are embedded in our daily sense-making (Malik, 2019). Additionally, if we have learned anything from and about stories, it is that they present themselves not only as worldviews but also as embodied feelings, shaping even our bodily reactions. This duality underscores, once again, that patriarchy is not a 'thing'—a floating entity controlling our behaviour—but, among other things, an incorporated way of being. Finally, it would be a delusion—and a fallacy—to believe we can combat male-chauvinistic narratives without providing alternative ones.

The conversation about alternative narratives often carries the danger of declaring success prematurely. In the context of the spectacularisation of violence (Binik, 2020; Mark, 1969, p. 14) and the increasing thematisation of violence against women, we may want to exercise caution. The burgeoning critical discourse—both academic and lay—does not automatically translate into awareness. There is not only the risk of misrecognising this phenomenon, where change and progressive thinking mask underlying forms of misogyny (Bourdieu, 1977), but also the emergence of subtle forms of reactionary discourse. The ridicule and trivialisation of masculinity change—for instance, manifesting in jokes and anecdotes, even within progressive groups—often lead us to disregard essential conversations about culture, discourse, and emotions. It may seem trivial or unimportant to address the primary socialisation of men or to discuss the stories children are exposed to. Yet, these discussions are anything but shallow or naïve.

In any case, the project of dismantling femicide-fostering narratives must account for their broader interconnectedness. Thinking ahead from this perspective implies not only considering the issue of gender but also the surrounding beliefs about other connected issues, such as justice, education, and institutions. This endeavour also means acknowledging our own complicity in these narratives. Male-chauvinistic stories are not "just propped up by cartoonish bad men who hoard the spoils of patriarchy. They're held dearly by the 'good' men as well: the woke brothers, the 'I'm on your side' dudes, the 'I'm a father to daughters and I'm appalled' dads" (Malik, 2019, p. 34). Complicities, fears of speaking out, and turning a blind eye are, indeed, part of the issues we must address. If these perpetrators are overachievers (Manne, 2020), it means that the social fabric as a whole contains these norms.

In hindsight, naming the issue of femicide as 'femicide' with a specific label has been undeniably a subversive strategy, part of the performative aspect of language itself. The act of claiming a topic into a field, delimiting its contours within a feminist logic, not only politicises experiences but also challenges patriarchal structures. It also helps us aggregate into a movement. This does not exclude a critical perspective on social movements, the co-option by the state (Bumiller, 2008), or the notion that merely naming and shaming perpetrators will automatically reduce the rates of violence (Boxall, 2024), or many other singular processes associated with the thematisation of femicide.

The discussion of femicide as an emergent field and topic has undoubtedly led to a conversation about resources, exposing the fact that this battle is not merely a superstructural debate about culture but also a material battle over resources. There is consensus that the majority of funding goes to victims/survivors, statistical registries, and campaigns. International organisations, which set funding priorities, often leave other facets unaddressed or delegitimised—such as, until recently, children of victims, or even today, strategies for dealing with perpetrators post-imprisonment. Ultimately, this reminds us of Weber's paradox of solving modern state problems with bureaucratic solutions: it creates further bureaucratic structures.

Things have undoubtedly begun to shift. In the context of what has been a profoundly troubling few years for violence against women, conversations have moved decisively towards holding men accountable while also addressing structural changes in masculinities. This aligns with arguments suggesting that, rather than relying solely on condemnation (such as through criminal laws), we need to foster alternative narratives and forms of subjectivity. Organisations like PROMUNDO and MenEngage promote initiatives such as tailored masculinities programmes and campaigns focused on engaged fatherhood that promote alternative emotional styles, acknowledgement of power structures and equitable interactions while challenging traditional gender norms. All these efforts point towards similar transformative pathways.

The bottom line is that to address an issue as layered and systemic as femicide, advocating for collective policies—ranging from upstream prevention strategies to targeted actions aimed at men—is essential. Transforming dominant narratives about intimate relationships, conflict, and gender is not optional but fundamental to ending femicides. Yet, this path may rely more on creating new bonds and narratives than merely destroying existing ones. As hooks (2004) eloquently states: "Only a revolution of values in our nation will end male violence, and that revolution will necessarily be based on a love ethic. To create loving men, we must love males" (p. 24).

On a Personal Note

> A revolution is precisely the effort to change the world through the transformation of the intellectual and moral structures. (Gramsci, 1971, p. 137)

I dedicated the majority of this book to understanding discourse: the words we use, the fables we hear, and the interpretations we form. From the outset, I suggested that femicide can appear as an almost amorphous phenomenon, heavily shaped by legal categories and contemporary theories. For the purposes of this book, I believe it is fruitful to draw on a social constructivist and epistemological perspectivism—as it provides a lens through which we can critique our worldviews. However, this should not be confused with trivial relativism. The emphasis on ideas does not erase the material reality at the heart of the issue: the death of women. It would be a fallacy to disconnect our material world from the narrative one. On the contrary, this book seeks to remind us that the material and the discursive are inseparably linked.

This interconnectedness becomes particularly evident when we consider the rise of reactionary discourses in the twenty-first century. It would be naïve to assume that the rise of right-wing, belligerent governments across the globe will not influence critical issues like femicide. Even if we find the claims of politicians like Donald Trump, Javier Milei, Jair Bolsonaro, or businessmen such as Elon Musk and Mark Zuckerberg—who advocate for the return of traditional masculinities—absurd or laughable, we cannot deny the impact of their discourse. Regardless of how geopolitically distant these narratives may seem, or how outlandish or seemingly incoherent they appear—as Foucault once described them, "Ubu-esque"—they will inevitably affect us.

While separating our analytical and personal views may sometimes be necessary to achieve clarity or push the boundaries of reflexivity, it is equally important to understand why and for whom we conduct research. With shrinking financial resources, the manipulation of academia's agenda, and increasing interventions in education and social policy driven by conservative governments, it should be clear that the discourses that enable these governments have direct and far-reaching consequences on everyday life.

Given this, can we continue to ignore the power of discourse, or must we confront the way it shapes the material reality of violence, inequality, and justice?

References

Abu-Lughod, L. (2008). *Writing women's worlds: Bedouin stories*. University of California Press.

Adichie, C. (2009, July). *The danger of the single story* [Broadcast]. https://www.ted.com/talks/chimamanda_ngozi_adichie_the_danger_of_a_single_story/transcript?language=es

Adinkrah, M. (2004). Witchcraft accusations and female homicide victimization in contemporary Ghana. *Violence against Women, 10*(4), 325–356. https://doi.org/10.1177/1077801204263419

Ahmed, S. (2004). *The cultural politics of emotion*. Edinburgh University Press.

Ahmed, S. (2021). *Complaint!* Duke University Press.

Alexievich, S. (2017). *The unwomanly face of war: An oral history of women in World War II*. Random House.

Alvelais, F., Pitaro, I., Wenck, J., & Becker, T. (2019). *"No Justice for Me". Femicide and Impunity in Bolivia*. https://hrp.law.harvard.edu/wp-content/uploads/2019/03/No-Justice-for-Me.pdf

Arendt, H. (2006). Eichmann in Jerusalem: A report on the banality of evil. In *Evil: A very short introduction*. Penguin.

Arendt, H. (2018). *On human condition*. The University of Chicago Press.

Arias Ortiz, E., Giambruno, C., Morduchowicz, A., & Pineda, B. (2024). *The state of education in Latin America and the Caribbean 2023*. Inter-American Development Bank. https://doi.org/10.18235/0005515

M. H. Di Marco, *Narratives of Femicide Perpetrators in Latin America*, https://doi.org/10.1007/978-3-031-97367-3

Atwood, M. (1996). *Alias Grace*. Rosetta Books.

Auyero, J., & Swiston, D. (2009). *Flammable: Environmental suffering in Argentine shantytown*. Oxford University Press.

Bancroft, L. (2003). *Why does he do that? Inside the minds of angry and controlling men*. Berkley Books.

Bancroft, L., Silverman, J., & Ritchie, D. (2011). *The batterer as parent: Addressing the impact of domestic violence on family dynamics*. Sage.

Bandelli, D. (2017). Femicide, gender and violence: Discourses and counterdiscourses in Italy. In *Femicide, gender and violence: Discourses and counterdiscourses in Italy*. Springer International Publishing. https://doi.org/10.1007/978-3-319-47785-5/COVER

Barán Attias, T. (2020). Víctimas de violencia sexual: Construcción de comunidades de creyentes y acceso a la(s) justicia(s). *Século XXI – Revista de Ciências Sociais, 9*(2), 415–445. https://doi.org/10.5902/2236672541166

Barrancos, D. (2023). *Historia mínima de los feminismos en América Latina*. Prometeo Editorial & El Colegio de México.

Becker, H. (1998). *Tricks of the trade: How to think about your research while you're doing it*. University of Chicago Press.

Benjamin, J. (1988). *The bonds of love: Psychoanalysis, feminism and the problem of domination*. Pantheon.

Berger, P., & Luckmann, T. (2017). *The social construction of reality*. Open Road Media.

Berggren, K., & Gottzén, L. (2022). Rethinking male peer support theory: Social network responses to young men's violence against women. *The Journal of Men's Studies, 30*(2), 291–307. https://doi.org/10.1177/10608265211068013

Berggren, K., Gottzén, L., & Bornäs, H. (2021). Theorising masculinity and intimate partner violence. In L. Gottzén, M. Bjørnholt, & F. Boonzaier (Eds.), *Men, mascunities and intimate partner violence* (pp. 34–51). Routledge.

Binik, O. (2020). *The fascination with violence in contemporary society. When crime is sublime*. Springer.

Bird, S. (1996). Welcome to the men's club: Homosociality and the maintenance of hegemonic masculinity. *Gender and Society, 10*(2), 120–132.

Bourdieu, P. (1977). *Outline of a theory of practice*. Cambridge University Press.

Bourdieu, P. (2017). The biographical illusion. In *Biography in theory* (pp. 210–216). De Gruyter.

Bourgois, P. (2003). *In search of respect: Selling crack in El Barrio (structural analysis in the social sciences)*. Cambridge University Press.

Boxall, H. (2024, July 23). Naming and shaming domestic violence perpetrators doesn't work to keep women safe. Here's why. *The Conversation.*

Brown, M. (2013). Penal spectatorship and the culture of punishment. In D. Scott (Ed.), *Why prison?* (pp. 108–124). Cambridge University Press.

Bruner, J. (1990). *Acts of meaning*. Harvard University Press.

Bruner, J. (2002). *Making stories: Law, literature, life*. Farrar, Strauss and Giroux.

Brunke, L. I., & Boira, S. (2021). Legal codification without justice: Causes and manifestations of impunity in Latin American cases of femicide. *Verfassung und Recht in Übersee/law and Politics in Africa, Asia and Latin America, 54*(4), 485–507.

Bumiller, K. (2008). *In an abusive state: How neoliberalism appropriated the feminist movement against sexual violence*. Duke University Press Books.

Bunn, R. (2023). Critical narratives or crime stories? The ethics and politics of narrative research in criminology. *The British Journal of Criminology, 63*(6), 1557–1573. https://doi.org/10.1093/BJC/AZAC101

Burke, K. (1969). *Grammar of motives*. University of California Press.

Burns, A. (2018). *Milkman*. Faber & Faber.

Butler, J. (2005). *Giving an account of oneself*. Fordham University Press.

Butler, J. (2006). *Gender Trouble. Feminism and the Subversion of Identity*. Routledge.

Carrère, E. (2024). *V13. Chronicle of a trial*. Farrer, Straus and Giroux.

Carrión, L. (2018). *La fosa de agua. Desapariciones y feminicidios en el Río de los Remedios*. Debate.

Cassino, D., & Besen-Cassino, Y. (2021). *Gender threat: American masculinity in the face of change*. Stanford University Press.

Chaitin, J. (2004). My story, my life, my identity. *International Journal of Qualitative Methods, 3*(4), 1–15. https://doi.org/10.1177/160940690400300401

Christie, N. (1981). *Limits to pain*. Universitetsforlaget.

Cohen, S., & Wills, T. A. (1985). Stress, social support, and the buffering hypothesis. *Psychological Bulletin, 98*(2), 310–357. https://doi.org/10.1037/0033-2909.98.2.310

Cole, S., & Phillips, L. (2008). The violence against women campaigns in Latin America. *Feminist Criminology, 3*(2), 145–168. https://doi.org/10.1177/1557085108317139

Connell, R., & Messerschmidt, J. (2005). Hegemonic masculinity: Rethinking the concept. *Gender & Society, 19*(6), 829–859. https://doi.org/10.1177/0891243205278639

Cooley, C. (2010). *Human nature and the social order*. Nabu Press.

Crewe, B. (2009). *The prisoner society: Power, adaptation and social life in an English prison*. Oxford University Press.

Crewe, B. (2020). The depth of imprisonment. *Punishment & Society, 23*(3), 335–354. https://doi.org/10.1177/1462474520952153

D'Ignazio, C. (2024). Counting feminicide. In *Counting feminicide*. The MIT Press.

Danto, A. C. (1994). *The transfiguration of commonplace: A philosophy of art*. Harvard University Press.

Dawson, M., & Mobated Vega, S. (Eds.). (2023). *The Routledge international handbook on femicide and feminicide*. Routledge.

DeKeseredy, W., & Schwartz, M. (2013). *Male peer support and violence against women: The history and verification of a theory*. University Press of New England.

Denzin, N. (1989). *Interpretative biography: Qualitative research methods*. Sage.

Devaney, J., Bradbury-Jones, C., Macy, R., Øverlien, C., & Holt, S. (2021). *Routledge international handbook of domestic violence and abuse*. Routledge.

Dheensa, S., Morgan, K., Love, B., & Cramer, H. (2022). Researching men's violence against women as feminist women researchers: The tensions we face. *Violence against Women, 30*(2), 347–371. https://doi.org/10.1177/10778012221134823

Di Marco, M. H., & Evans, D. P. (2020). Society, her or me? An explanatory model of intimate femicide among male perpetrators in Buenos Aires, Argentina. *Feminist Criminology, 15*(5).

Di Marco, M. H., & Rowlands, J. (2025). Beyond a naive enquiry into intimate partner femicide: Challenges, dilemmas, and opportunities in the study of perpetrators. In C. Borda-Niño-Wildman (Ed.), *Routledge international handbook of gender-based violence research*. Routledge/Taylor & Francis.

Di Marco, M. H., & Sandberg, S. (2024). Fear, helplessness, pain, anger: The narrated emotions of intimate femicide perpetrators in Latin America. *International Sociology, 39*(2).

Dobash, R. E., & Dobash, R. (2015). *When men murder women*. Oxford University Press.

Dobash, R. E., & Dobash, R. (2017). When women are murdered. In *The handbook of homicide* (pp. 131–148). Wiley Blackwell.

Douglas, M. (1992). *Risk and blame: Essays in cultural theory*. Routledge.

Douglas, M. (1997). The depoliticization of risk. In R. Ellis & M. Thompson (Eds.), *Culture matters: Essays in honor of Aaron Wildavsky* (pp. 121–132). Westview Press.

Elliott, D., & Wolf-Meyer, M. J. (Eds.). (2024). *Naked Fieldnotes: A rough guide to ethnographic writing*. University of Minnesota Press.

Enander, V., Krantz, G., Lysell, H., & Örmon, K. (2021). Before the killing: Intimate partner homicides in a process perspective, Part I. *Journal of Gender-Based Violence, 5*(1), 59–74. https://doi.org/10.1332/239868020X15922355479497

Espino, A. (2024). Historia de los movimientos feministas en América Latina. In M. Deciancio & J. Loza (Eds.), *Relaciones internacionales y feminismos: Voces latinoamericanas en un debate global* (pp. 182–204). Teseo.

Evans, D. P., Di Marco, M. H., Narasimhan, S., Maino Vieytes, M., Curran, A., & White, M. (2023). Male perpetrators' accounts of femicide: A global systematic review. In M. Dawson & S. Mobayed (Eds.), *The Routledge International Handbook on Femicide and Feminicide* (pp. 890–907). Routledge Handbooks.

Fahs, E., Di Marco, M. H., & Evans, D. P. (2023). "There was no other option": Femicide perpetrators' sensemaking on gender and violence in Buenos Aires, Argentina. *Gender and Society, 10*(1), 29–37. https://doi.org/10.1089/VIO.2021.0093

Farmer, P. (2009). On suffering and structural violence: A view from below. *Race/Ethnicity: Multidisciplinary Global Contexts, 3*(1), 11–28.

Feld, C., & Salvi, V. (Eds.). (2019). *Las Voces De La Represión: Declaraciones de perpetradores de la dictadura argentina*. Miño y Dávila editores.

Fernández, A. M. (2012). Femicidios: La ferocidad del patriarcado. *Nomadías,* 0(16), 47–73. https://doi.org/10.5354/0719-0905.2012.24957

Flood, M. (2007). Men, sex, and homosociality. *Men and Masculinities, 10*(3), 339–359. https://doi.org/10.1177/1097184X06287761

Foucault, M. (1990). *The history of sexuality, vol. 1: An introduction*. Vintage; Reissue edition.

Foucault, M. (2002). *The order of things—An archeology of the human sciences*. Psychology Press.

Frank, A. W. (1995). *The wounded storyteller: Body, illness, and ethics*(2nd ed.). University of Chicago Press.

Fransman, K., & Plackett, J. (2021). *Gender swapped fairy tales*. Faber & Faber.

Freud, S. (1977). The dynamics of transference. In R. J. Langs (Ed.), *Classics in psychoanalytic technique* (pp. 3–8). Jason Aronson.

Fujii, L. A. (2010). Shades of truth and lies: Interpreting testimonies of war and violence. *Journal of Peace Research, 47*(2), 231–241.

Garfinkel, H. (1967). *Studies in ethnometodology*. Prentice-Hall.

Garland, D. (2003). The rise of risk. In R. V. Ericson & A. Doyle (Eds.), *Risk and morality* (pp. 1–10). University of Toronto Press.

Geertz, C. (1973). *The interpretation of cultures*. Basic Books.

Gergen, K. (1991). *The saturated self: Dilemmas of identity in contemporary life*. Basic Books.

Gergen, K. (1994). *Realities and relationships: Soundings in social construction*. Harvard University Press.

Giddens, A. (1984). *The constitution of society*. University of California Press.

Gnisci, A., & Pace, A. (2016). Lethal domestic violence as a sequential process: Beyond the traditional regression approach to risk factors. *Current Sociology, 64*(7), 1108–1123. https://doi.org/10.1177/0011392116629809

Goffman, E. (1956). *The presentation of self in everyday life*. Doubleday.

Gottzén, L. (2019). Chafing masculinity: Heterosexual violence and young men's shame. *Feminism & Psychology, 29*(2), 286–302. https://doi.org/10.1177/0959353518776341

Goussinsky, R., & Yassour-Borochowitz, D. (2012). "I killed her, but I never laid a finger on her"—A phenomenological difference between wife-killing and wife-battering. *Aggression and Violent Behavior, 17*(6), 553–564. https://doi.org/10.1016/j.avb.2012.07.009

Gramsci, A. (1971). *Selections from the prison notebooks*. International Publishers.

Guillemin, M., & Gillam, L. (2004). Ethics, reflexivity, and "ethically important moments" in research. *Qualitative Inquiry, 10*(2), 261–280. https://doi.org/10.1177/1077800403262360

Gusfield, J. R. (1984). *The culture of public problems: Drinking-driving and the symbolic order*. University of Chicago Press.

Haines, S., Poo, A.-J., & Strozzi-Heckler, R. (2019). *The politics of trauma: Somatics, healing, and social*. North Atlantic Books.

Halberstam, J. (2011). *The queer art of failure*. Duke University Press.

Hearn, J. (1998). *The violences of men: How men talk about and how agencies respond to men's violence to women*. Sage.

Hearn, J., Aavik, K., Collinson, D. L., & Thym, A. (2025). Studying men, masculinities, organizations and organizing: Introducing the Handbook. In J. Hearn, K. Aavik, D. L. Collinson, & A. Thym (Eds.), *Routledge handbook on men, masculinities and organizations: Theories, practices and futures of organizing* (pp. 1–20). Routledge.

Hemingway, E. (2006). *The sun also rises*. Simon & Schuster USA.

Hochschild, A. R. (1979). Work, feeling rules, and social structure. *American Journal of Sociology, 85*(3), 551–575.

Hooks, B. (2004). *The will to change: Men, masculinity, and change*. Washington Square Press Inc.

Husseini, R. (2009). *Murder in the name of honour: The true story of one woman's heroic fight against an unbelievable crime*. Oneworld Publications.

Illouz, E. (2013). *Why love hurts: A sociological explanations*. Wiley John & Sons.

Johnson, H., Eriksson, L., Mazerolle, P., & Wortley, R. (2019). Intimate femicide: The role of coercive control. *Feminist Criminology, 14*(1), 3–23. https://doi.org/10.1177/1557085117701574

Johnson, N. (2000). *'The right to have rights': Gender politics, citizenship and the state in Uruguay* [PhD Dissertation]. Queen Mary and Westfield College.

Josselson, R. (2009). The present of the past: Dialogues with memory over time. *Journal of Personality, 77*(3), 647–668. https://doi.org/10.1111/J.1467-6494.2009.00560.X

Kimmel, M. (2019). Targeting women. In *Angry white men: American masculinity at the end of an era* (pp. 169–198). Bold Type Books.

Kohan, J. (2021). Femicidios en la Argentina en el período 2002–2018: ¿fenómeno en alza o visibilización de un antiguo problema? *Notas e Población, 112*, 161–189.

Kruse, A. E., & Skilbrei, M. L. (2024). The monster and the self: Taking on the monstrosity of sexual violations. *Punishment and Society, 26*(5), 840–859. https://doi.org/10.1177/14624745231221933

Labov, W., & Waletzky, J. (1997). Narrative analysis: Oral version of personal experience. *Journal of Narrative and Life History, 7*(1–4), 3–38.

Lacan, J. (1973). *The four fundamental concepts of psychoanalysis*. Le Seuil.

Lagarde y de los Ríos, M. (2012). *El feminismo en mi vida. Hitos, claves y topías*. Instituto de las Mujeres.

Lagarde, M. (2006). Del femicidio al feminicidio. *Desde El Jardín de Freud, 0*(6), 216–225.

Lakoff, G., & Johnson, M. (1981). *Metaphors we live by*. University of Chicago Press.

Lawrence-Lightfoot, S. (1997). *The art and science of portraiture*. Jossey-Bass.

Malik, N. (2019). *We need new stories: The myths that subvert freedom*. Weidenfeld & Nicolson.

Manne, K. (2017). *Down girl. The logic of misogyny*. Oxford University Press.

Manne, K. (2020). *Entitled: How male privilege hurts women*. Crown.

Mannheim, K. (1991). *Ideology and utopia*. Routledge.

Mark, K. (1969). *Marx/Engels selected works*. Progress Publishers.

Marx, K. (1977). *A contribution to the critique of political economy*. Progress Publishers.

Mathews, S., Jewkes, R., & Abrahams, N. (2011). "I had a hard life": Exploring childhood adversity in the shaping of masculinities among men who killed an intimate partner in South Africa. *British Journal of Criminology, 51*(6), 960–977. https://doi.org/10.1093/bjc/azr051

Mathews, S., Jewkes, R., & Abrahams, N. (2015). "So now i'm the man": Intimate partner femicide and its interconnections with expressions of masculinities in South Africa. *British Journal of Criminology, 55*(1), 107–124. https://doi.org/10.1093/bjc/azu076

McGee Deutsch, S. (1991). Gender and sociopolitical change in twentieth-century Latin America. *Hispanic American Historical Review, 71*(2), 259–306. https://doi.org/10.1215/00182168-71.2.259

McKibben, E., & Breheny, M. (2023). Making sense of making sense of time: Longitudinal narrative research. *International Journal of Qualitative Methods*. https://doi.org/10.1177/16094069231160928

Melo, P. (2023). *The simple art of killing a woman*. Restless Books.

Menéndez, E. L. (2008). Epidemiología sociocultural: Propuestas y posibilidades. *Región y Sociedad*, *XX*(2), 5–50.

Messerschmidt, J. (2000). *Nine lives: Adolescent masculinities, the body, and violence*. Westview Press.

Moriconi Bezerra, M. (2013). *Ser violento. Los orígenes de la inseguridad y la víctima-cómplice*. Capital Intelectual.

Noel, G. (2011). Algunos dilemas éticos del trabajo antropológico con actores implicados en actividades delictivas. *Ankulegi, 15*, 127–140.

Noel, G., & Garriga Zucal, J. (2010). Notas para una definición antropológica de la violencia: un debate en curso. *PUBLICAR-En Antropología y Ciencias Sociales, 0*(9), 97–121.

Oddone, C. (2017). Poner el foco en los hombres para eliminar la violencia contra las mujeres. *Revista CIDOB d'Afers Internacionals, 117*, 145–169. https://doi.org/10.24241/rcai.2017.117.3.145

Orwell, G. (1941). *All art is propaganda*. Mariner Books Classics.

Orwell, G. (1978). *Decline of the English Murder*. Penguin.

Palacios, R. (2016). *Conchita. Ricardo Barreda, el hombre que no amaba a las mujeres*. Planeta.

Pasinato, W., & de Ávila, T. P. (2022). Criminalization of femicide in Latin America: Challenges of legal conceptualization. *Current Sociology, 71*(1), 60–77. https://doi.org/10.1177/00113921221090252

Plummer, K. (1995). *Telling Sexual Stories: Power*. Routledge.

Plummer, K. (2019). *Narrative power: The struggle for human value*. Polity.

Posey, B. M. (2023). Black femicides matter: Conceptualizing the killings of black girls and women as structural and cultural violence. *Homicide Studies, 28*, 313–340. https://doi.org/10.1177/10887679231209227

Presser, L. (2013). *Why we harm*. Rutgers University Press.

Presser, L. (2022). *Unsaid: Analyzing harmful silences*. University of California Press.

Presser, L., & Sandberg, S. (2015). Introduction. What is the story? In *Narrative criminology: Understanding stories of crime* (pp. 1–20). NYU Press.

Pridemore, W. A. (2007). Change and stability in the characteristics of homicide victims, offenders and incidents during rapid social change. *The British Journal of Criminology, 47*(2), 331–345. https://doi.org/10.1093/BJC/AZL029

Regis-Moura, A., Ferreira, L. B., Bonfá-Araujo, B., & Iglesias, F. (2021). "If not mine, she won't belong to another": Mechanisms of moral disengagement in a femicide perpetrator from Brazil. *Violence against Women, 28*(12–13), 3135–3153. https://doi.org/10.1177/10778012211038969

Renehan, N. (2021). Facilitators of probation-based domestic violence perpetrator programmes: 'Who's in the room?' *Probation Journal, 68*(3), 310–329. https://doi.org/10.1177/02645505211025083

Restrepo, L. (2018). *Los divinos*. Alfaguara.

Reyes, D. (2019). *Cometierra*. Sigilo Editorial.

Riches, D. (1986). The phenomenon of violence. In D. Riches (Ed.), *Anthropology of violence* (pp. 1–27). Blackwell.

Ricœur, P. (2004). *Memory, history, forgetting*. University of Chicago Press.

Riemann, G. (2006). An introduction to "doing biographical research." *Historical Social Research, 31*(3), 6–28.

Rivera Garza, C. (2021). *El invencible verano de Liliana*. Penguin Random House.

Robben, A. (1996). The politics of truth and emotion among victims and perpetrators of violence. In C. Nordstrom & A. Robben (Eds.), *Fieldwork under fire: Contemporary studies of violence and culture* (pp. 81–104). University of California Press.

Robben, A. (2014). Ethnographic seduction, transference, and resistance in dialogues about terror and violence in Argentina. *Ethos, 24*(1), 71–106.

Robben, A., & Hinton, A. (2023). *Perpetrators: Encountering humanity's dark side*. Stanford University Press.

Rosaldo, M. (1994). Towards an anthropology of self and feeling. In R. A. Shweder & R. A. LeVine (Eds.), *Culture theory: Essays on mind, self, and emotion* (pp. 137–157). Cambridge University Press.

Rose, J. (2021). *On violence and on violence against women*. Farrar, Straus and Giroux.

Rosenthal, G. (2004). Biographical research. In C. Seale, G. Gobo, J. F. Gubrium, & D. Silverman (Eds.), *Qualitative research practice* (pp. 49–65). Sage. https://doi.org/10.4135/9781848608191.d7

Rosenthal, G. (2010). The holocaust in three generations: families of victims and perpetrators of the Nazi Regime. In *2003*. Barbara Budrich Publishers.

Rosenthal, G. (2018). Biographical research and case reconstruction. In *Interpretive social research—An introduction* (pp. 155–189). Universitätsverlag Göttingen.

Ruggiero, K. (2001). Passion, perversity, and the pace of justice in Argentina at the turn of the last century. In R. Salvatore, C. Aguirre, & G. Joseph (Eds.), *Crime and punishment in Latin America: Law and society since late colonial times* (pp. 211–232). Duke University Press.

Rumpf, T., Horn, S., Vogt, C., Göbel, K., Görgen, T., Zibulski, K. M., Uttenweiler, V., & Bondü, R. (2024). Leaking in intimate partner homicide: A systematic review. *Trauma, Violence & Abuse, 25*(4). https://doi.org/10.1177/15248380241237213

Russell, D. (1976). *Report on the international tribunal on crimes against women*. https://www.dianarussell.com/f/Crimes_Against_Women_Tribunal.pdf

Ryan, W. (1971). *Blaming the victim*. Pantheon Books.

Sandberg, S. (2010). What can "lies" tell us about life? Notes towards a framework of narrative criminology. *Journal of Criminal Justice Education, 21*(4), 447–465. https://doi.org/10.1080/10511253.2010.516564

Sandberg, S., Tutenges, S., & Copes, H. (2015). Stories of violence: A narrative criminological study of ambiguity. *British Journal of Criminology, 55*(6), 1168–1186. https://doi.org/10.1093/bjc/azv032

Sanjek, R. (2004). Going public: Responsibilities and strategies in the aftermath of ethnography. *Human Organization, 63*(4), 444–456. https://doi.org/10.17730/HUMO.63.4.MUD4GJB5MDV69YBA

Sapriza, G. (2015). "Nos habíamos amado tanto". Años revueltos. Mujeres, colectivos y la pelea por el espacio público. *Revista Estudos Feministas, 23*(3), 939–958. https://www.redalyc.org/pdf/381/38142136015.pdf

Saramago, J. (2000). *The tale of the unknown Island*. Harpervia.

Scheper-Hughes, N. (1992). Nervoso: Medicine, sickness and human needs. In *Death without weeping: The violence of everyday life in Brazil* (pp. 167–215). University of California Press.

Scheper-Hughes, N. (1995). The primacy of the ethical: Propositions for a militant anthropology. *Current Anthropology, 36*(3), 409–440. https://doi.org/10.2979/HISTMEMO.31.1.0059

Scheper-Hughes, N. (1997). Demography without numbers. In D. Kertzer & T. Fricke (Eds.), *Anthropological demography: Toward a new synthesis* (pp. 201–222). University of Chicago Press.

Schulman, S. (1984). *The Sophie Horowitz story*. Naiad Press.

Schultze, M. (2012). *Siempre será después*. Alfaguara.

Schutz, A. (1967). *The problem of social reality: Collected papers I*. Nijhoff.

Sedgwick, E. K. (1985). *Between men: English literature and male homosocial desire*. Columbia University Press.

Segato, R. (2003). *Las estructuras elementales de la violencia. Ensayos sobe género entre la antropología, el psicoanálisis y los derechos humanos*. Universidad Nacional de Quilmes.

Segato, R. (2016). *La guerra contra las mujeres*. Traficantes de sueños. https://doi.org/10.35305/rpu.v0i3.42

Segato, R. (2024). *War against women*. Polity Press.

Shuman, A. (2010). *Other people's stories: Entitlement claims and the critique of empathy*. University of Illinois Press.

Sinclair, V., & Steinkoler, M. (2018). *On psychoanalysis and violence: Contemporary Lacanian perspectives*. Routledge.

Smith, P. (2005). *Why war? The cultural logic of Iraq, the Gulf War, and Suez*. University of Chicago Press.

Sontag, S. (2003). *Regarding the pain of others*. Picador/Farrar, Straus and Giroux.

Stanko, E. A., & Hobdell, K. (1993). Assault on men: Masculinity and male victimization. *The British Journal of Criminology, 33*(3), 400–415. https://doi.org/10.1093/OXFORDJOURNALS.BJC.A048333

Suárez Val, H., D'Ignazio, C., Acosta Romero, J., Teng, M. Q., & Fumega, S. (2023). Data artivism and feminicide. *Big Data and Society, 10*(2). https://doi.org/10.1177/20539517231215356/ASSET/IMAGES/LARGE/10.1177_20539517231215356-FIG3.JPEG

Svampa, M. (2000). Identidades astilladas. De la Patria Metalúrgica al Heavy Meta. In *Desde Abajo. LA transformación de las identidades sociales* (pp. 106–136). Biblos.

Tewksbury, R., & Gagné, P. (2001). Assumed and presumed identities: Problems of self-presentation in field research. In *Extreme methods: Innovative approaches to Social Science research* (pp. 72–93). Allyn & Bacon.

UNODC, & UN Women. (2024). *Femicides in 2023: Global estimates of intimate partner/family member femicides*. https://www.unwomen.org/sites/default/files/2024-11/femicides-in-2023-global-estimates-of-intimate-partner-family-member-femicides-en.pdf

UNWomen, & UNODC. (2022). *International statistical framework for measuring gender-related killings of women and girls*.

Verkko, J. (1951). *Homicides and suicides in Finland and their dependence on national character*. G. E. C. Gads Forlag.

Viveros-Vigoya, M. (2016). Masculinities in the continuum of violence in Latin America. *Feminist Theory, 17*(2), 229–237. https://doi.org/10.1177/1464700116645879

Wacquant, L. J. D. (1989). Towards a reflexive sociology: A workshop with Pierre Bourdieu. *Sociological Theory, 7*(1), 26–63.

Walby, S., & Shire, K. (2024). *Trafficking chains: Modern slavery in society*. Modern Slavery in Society.

Walklate, S., & Fitz-Gibbon, K. (2023). Re-imagining the measurement of femicide: From 'thin' counts to 'thick' counts. *Current Sociology, 71*(1), 28–42. https://doi.org/10.1177/00113921221082698/ASSET/IMAGES/LARGE/10.1177_00113921221082698-FIG2.JPEG

Websdale, N. (2009). *Familicidal hearts: The emotional styles of 211 killers*. Oxford University Press.

West, C., & Zimmerman, D. H. (1987). Doing gender. *Gender and Society, 1*(2), 125–151.

Whynacht, A. (2019). *Insurgent love. Abolition and domestic homicide*. Fernwood Publishing.

Winch, P. (2018). *The idea of a social science and its relation to philosophy*. Routledge.

Witte, N. (2016). Palestinian voices from Haif. In G. Rosenthal (Ed.), *Established and outsiders at the same time: Self-images and we-images of Palestinians in the West Bank and in Israel* (pp. 159–180). Göttingen University Press.

Wittgenstein, L. (2009). *Philosophical investigations*. Wiley-Blackwell.

Wittgestein, L. (2021). *Tractatus logico-philosophicus*. Edinburgh University Press.

Worsley, L. (2014). *The art of the English murder*. Pegasus Crime.

Wright Mills, C. (1940). Situated action and vocabularies of motive. *American Sociological Review, 5*(6), 904–913.

Zerubavel, E. (2018). *Taken for granted: The remarkable power of the unremarkable*. Princeton University Press.

Index

M. H. Di Marco, *Narratives of Femicide Perpetrators in Latin America*, https://doi.org/10.1007/978-3-031-97367-3

www.ingramcontent.com/pod-product-compliance
Lightning Source LLC
Chambersburg PA
CBHW051413031125
34911CB00002B/70
* 9 7 8 3 0 3 1 9 7 3 6 6 6 *